NEW LIGHT
ON
DEPRESSION

This letter of condolence was written by President Abraham Lincoln to Fanny McCullough, the daughter of William McCullough, whom Lincoln had known well. When Fanny was a child, the future president had held her and her sister Nanny on his knees. Mutual friends informed the president of Fanny's depression over her father's death in a Civil War battle near Coffeeville, Mississippi, on December 5, 1862.[1] Only five days after Burnside's Union forces had received a crushing blow in the Battle of Fredericksburg, the President of the United States took the time to try to comfort his young friend, possibly because Lincoln knew the gloom of depression, having struggled with it personally for years. This great man evidently felt an obligation to set aside affairs of state long enough to shine a ray of light into the darkness of a young girl's hurting heart.

Knowing depression personally has caused many, including us, to embrace the calling to comfort others in distress with the comfort that we ourselves have experienced (see 2 Cor. 1:3–7). In this there is hope, purpose, meaning, and ultimately a joy that nothing can take away. We trust this book will encourage some to sense a similar calling while enabling them to fulfill it.

New Light on Depression

ON

Depression

HELP, HOPE, & ANSWERS
—— *for the* ——
DEPRESSED & THOSE WHO LOVE THEM

DAVID B. BIEBEL, D.MIN. &
HAROLD G. KOENIG, M.D.

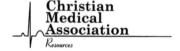

Christian
Medical
Association
Resources

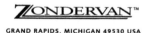

ZONDERVAN™

GRAND RAPIDS, MICHIGAN 49530 USA

ZONDERVAN™

New Light on Depression
Copyright © 2004 by David B. Biebel and Harold G. Koenig

Requests for information should be addressed to:

Zondervan, *Grand Rapids, Michigan 49530*

Library of Congress Cataloging-in-Publication Data

Biebel, David B.
    New light on depression : help, hope, and answers for the depressed and those who
love them / David B. Biebel, Harold G. Koenig.
        p. cm.
    Includes bibliographical references and index.
    ISBN 0-310-24729-2
    1. Depression, Mental—Religious aspects—Christianity. 2. Depression, Mental.
3. Depressed persons—Religious life. I. Koenig, Harold George. II. Title.
BV4910.34.B54 2004
248.8'625—dc22

        2003018784

Interior design by Beth Shagene

Printed in the United States of America

05 06 07 08 09 /❖ DC/ 10 9 8 7 6 5 4 3 2

Dear God:

We dedicate this book to all our fellow travelers on the journey called "depression" and those who care about or for us. May their faith be strengthened, their love deepened, and their hope increased by the words that follow. As this prayer is answered, our labors with depression and your labors to produce in us enough informed, compassionate sensitivity to become their journey-mates will not have been in vain.

David B. Biebel
Harold G. Koenig
Easter 2003

Disclaimer

This book, though biblically sound and medically reliable, is not intended to replace medical advice and/or evaluation that is best provided by a trained professional. Any medical or technical information, advice, or instruction is intended for the benefit of our readers without any guarantee with respect to results they may experience with regard to the same. Implementation of any information or advice in this book is the decision of the reader and at his or her own risk.

Explanation of Voices

When we say "we," we are speaking with one voice, in agreement. The use of the first person, "I," occurs from time to time, especially when we share from personal experience. In each case we use the author's initials (DB or HK) early in the segment to identify whom is speaking.

Explanation of Stories

Unless otherwise indicated, the stories in this book are true, though in most cases details have been changed to protect the privacy of the people involved. In all cases in which real names appear, they do so with permission of the persons involved.

Contents

Foreword

I have a relative who has battled depression. For many years, it drained her energy and, like a ball and chain, inhibited her from walking through life with confidence and joy. It was like she wore dark glasses that hid the vibrant colors of loving relationships and the experiences of everyday life. The world most days was a dull, dreary gray, and she lived with inner storms of anger punctuated by lighting bolts of emotional pain.

Her husband stood by her through it all. He helped her get the counseling and medication she needed. These things helped, but it was only in the last few years that she markedly improved, after she and those around her discovered what you are about to learn: depression is a whole-person disorder with biological, psychological, social, and spiritual roots. Addressing only one or two of them does not solve the problem. And there is no one magic cure.

A comprehensive, reliable, easy-to-read, and practical Christian book on depression is long overdue. You are now holding that resource in your hands. Rather than endorsing one view on depression and its treatment, the authors take a far-ranging, inclusive approach. They discuss the wide variety of counseling approaches and medical treatments objectively, even presenting examples of dialogues between counselors and patients. They cover both Christian and secular counseling approaches and include less-well-known techniques that hold promise.

More important, they have written in easily understood language and from the valuable perspectives of both physician and pastor. You won't have to wade through jargon or unexplained medical terminology to learn what you need to know.

The authors advocate a multidisciplinary team approach tailored to the true needs of the depressed person. They emphasize the critical importance of greater cooperation among the religious and medical experts who provide treatment and counseling.

The chapter on myths and misconceptions is, alone, worth the price of the book. Among other things, the authors dispel the belief that real Christians don't become depressed. Denying that your depression is real only worsens symptoms and delays treatment, or makes it impossible to deal with.

Most important, the authors help you learn how to live with depression and help you realize that it can bring growth and a new understanding of grace.

As a physician, I've taken care of many patients with depression and read widely on the topic. This is the best resource I've ever seen. Get ready for large doses of insight, gripping stories, and practical suggestions. The darkness of depression in your life, or in the life of someone you care about, is about to be pierced by *New Light on Depression*.

David Stevens, M.D.
Executive Director
The Christian Medical
    and Dental Associations

Acknowledgments

We wish to thank:

Dr. Gene Rudd, Associate Executive Director of the Christian Medical and Dental Associations, for entrusting this project to us.

Cindy Hays Lambert, Zondervan acquisitions editor, for shepherding the project through all its various stages, because she believed its message and ministry were crucial.

Traci Mullins, whose editing was at first painful, but "painful are the wounds of a friend."

Dr. Steve Mory, who began as our reviewer and ended up our friend and a significant contributor to what follows.

All our other fellow pilgrims, some named and some anonymous or with identities disguised, who interacted with our ideas and allowed us to use their thoughts and sometimes their stories. This book would not be the same without their contributions.

DEPRESSION, A MANY FACTORED THING

CHAPTER 1

Like Nailing Jell-O to the Wall

Some people see depression as the designer disorder of our age, implying that this disorder somehow became more prevalent with the introduction of effective medications to treat it. Prozac, an antidepressant that helped vault depression into prominence a few years ago, is so well-known there are jokes about it. Yet behind the laughter, for many, the biblical proverb is true: "Even in laughter the heart may be in pain" (Prov. 14:13 NASB).

The truth is that depression is as old as humanity, at least since Adam and Eve were driven from their place of perfect peace. In what may be the Bible's oldest portion, Job, the paragon of patience, says, "Sighing comes to me instead of food; my groans pour out like water. What I feared has come upon me; what I dreaded has happened to me. I have no peace, no quietness; I have no rest, but only turmoil" (Job 3:24–26). Obviously, depression is no respecter of faith—affecting believers and unbelievers alike.

Depression is also no respecter of persons, as it afflicts politicians and world leaders, recipients of various prestigious awards, athletes, authors, actors, musicians . . . and garden-variety folk like you and us. It affected Sarah, as follows in her own words:

"By my late thirties," she writes, "I had suffered a series of losses over a period of a few years, and though I had grieved, I believed I had weathered the losses well. After years of struggling with infertility, I had conceived, only to lose my unborn child through miscarriage in the fourth month. The grief was deep and painful, but I was not debilitated by it. In fact, I experienced newfound strength in the wake of it as my faith sustained me. Then a near-adoption of two adorable little preschool sisters ended abruptly when the birthmother changed her mind.

"A few years later, to our delight, my husband and I adopted a nine-year-old boy who had known great loss and trauma in his own short life. A few months later I conceived again, this time ending in a ruptured tubal pregnancy that almost took my life. There were new waves of grief, but once again I also felt inner strength and resolve. I felt God's power in very tangible ways and knew that God would weave the grief into my life in healing ways.

"Within a short time, we began to experience major upheaval as we tried to help our son forge a new life for himself. We had expected this, given his prior life events, but it still stretched us in every way. I loved being a mom, though I also experienced the drain and discouragement of realizing that all the love in the world for our son could not meet his deepest needs. In his young adolescent years we watched in pain and the worst kind of helplessness as our son descended into a life of drug abuse. As we struggled to anchor him through this time, one of his birthparents swept back into our lives, which sent our son into a tailspin. At the tender age of fifteen he left us to live with this birthparent, dropped out of high school, and adopted the chaotic lifestyle of drugs and poverty. This was a new kind of grief and loss that lacked the resolution of my earlier losses, leaving me feeling empty and hollow, dejected and demoralized. I was grieving deeply, but my faith was secure.

"A year later I was still filled with intense sadness and having some difficulties managing anxiety, but I did not consider myself depressed. I was grieving, and grieving hurts. I was also worrying for my husband, whose grief was deep but beyond my reach to help. I did realize, however, that I had lost a sense of knowing what 'normal' was. I felt I was emotionally limping.

"Then we sold the business we had nurtured together for nearly two decades and took positions at a company in another state, leaving behind our home church, close extended family, and lifelong friends. The new job did not turn out to be what I had expected. I found myself in a company embroiled in internal struggle and the upheaval of major changes in philosophy and mission—coming apart at the seams.

"My anxiety level became toxic. I became unable to eat or sleep, fearful of getting out of bed and facing the day. I felt guilty for being so weak and ashamed that I felt like I was falling apart. At work, others perceived me as all together because I hid my fears, but at times I was unable to stop trembling, my heart pounded, and my breathing was labored. By the time I got home from work, I just wanted to curl up on the sofa with a pillow and blanket and watch television, hoping for sleep to come. I couldn't rest or relax—all I felt was turmoil and stress, anxiety and darkness.

"In retrospect I can see the depression clearly, but at the time I was blind to it. All I saw was that I was weak and filled with worry—and I felt guilty about both. It did not occur to me to see a medical doctor. I was sure my coping problem was due to my emotional weakness and was actually failure. So I kept trying to talk myself into being stronger and getting myself through this, while berating myself for not being able to pull out of it.

"All the previous losses in my life resurfaced, and I grieved them again. All my former support systems—long-term friends, home church, extended family—were many miles away. Eventually, I concluded that I needed help with the anxiety, while at the same time feeling too over-whelmed to try to find a counselor. I was certain the problem was all in my head, and I felt ashamed of that. I simply could not muster the strength and energy to search for a counselor, and I felt guilty about that as well. I was caught in a negative cycle that I couldn't seem to break.

"Then I learned I needed surgery, which turned out to be a blessing in disguise. My wise surgeon recognized my depression and anxiety and sent me to a new primary care physician. I'll never forget that first visit as 'the light went on' when the doctor asked a series of questions: How was I sleeping? How was my appetite? How was work going? What was I doing that I enjoyed? I recognized these as classic questions about depression. How had I missed this in myself? By the time she finished asking her questions, I already knew the answer. I was clinically depressed.

"Then she explained that, no matter what had brought on this depression, it had become a biological problem that needed biological treatment. She recommended medication immediately.

"I had mixed reactions to taking an antidepressant, though. I did *not* want to turn to pills just because I couldn't handle life's problems, and I was afraid of developing a dependency on them. I had always sought to understand myself and to rise to every challenge with God as my strength. Would this be a cop-out? Would it be escape instead of heal-ing? Would I only be masking deeper problems? Shouldn't my faith be enough to sustain me?

"Yet I was desperate and I knew it. Though fearful of the medication and its implications, I was more fearful of the darkness inside that was smothering my ability to function. And I did hear the voice of God in the calm voice of reason from my doctor. Her words, reinforced by a few wise friends and family, helped ease my concerns. I agreed to treat my medically depressed condition just as I was treating my body with its need for surgery. Something was in need of repair, and it only made sense to treat it. I began the medication the same week I had my surgery."

There's Nothing Easy about Depression

Have you personally struggled with depression or tried to help someone mired in what John Bunyan, author of *Pilgrim's Progress*, called the "slough of despond" (the muck of despair)? If so, you can surely identify with some of the feelings Sarah expresses: pain mixed with faith, drained and discouraged, helpless, empty, dejected, anxious, fearful, guilty, ashamed, needing to hide, exhausted, immersed in and smothered by darkness, weak, feeling like a failure, isolated and lonely, overwhelmed, stuck, confused, torn, desperate, immobilized, having lost a sense of normalcy. You also already know that there is nothing easy about this disorder. Regardless of what some experts may claim, it's not easy to understand depression's causes and cures or to comprehend the myriad masks it wears. Only those who have experienced depression personally can imagine its ability to thoroughly permeate a person's life, stealing whatever joy existed and replacing it with murkiness and pain.

In addition to these challenges, a most daunting task is to define what we mean when we use the term *depression*. Were you to ask people on the street to define it, you might hear words like "sad," "the blues," or "down in the dumps." Nearly everyone you might ask would offer some description, though, because depression happens to most everyone at some time in their life.

The word *depression* is used in navigation to mean the angular distance of a celestial object below the horizon. In geology, a depression is a low point or hollow. The Stock Market crash of 1929 led to what in the United States became known as the Great Depression and contributed to a general worldwide economic depression. Surely during this dark period in history, many individuals suffered deeply with the disorder called depression. Yet to say that during the Great Depression many people were depressed is to sound like President Calvin Coolidge, who once said, "When large numbers of men are unable to find work, unemployment results."

Were you to ask a group of counselors to define depression, you might hear words like "mood disorder" or "psychiatric condition," but many of the terms you'd hear would classify or describe depression rather than define it. You might also hear questions, depending on their points of view, such as, "Are we talking about 'situational depression,' 'biological depression,' 'developmental depression,' or 'spiritual depression'?" and "Is it serious enough to be labeled a 'clinical' or 'major' depression?" From some you might hear terms connected with their theories of depression's causes, stating that depression is, for example, "a natural reaction to stress," "frozen rage," "repressed grudges," or even "unresolved guilt." Isn't it interesting how one word can have so many nuances of meanings? Speaking metaphorically, nailing down a definition of depression is like trying to nail psychological Jell-O to a wall.

Our preference is to keep it simple: *Depression is a state of existence marked by a sense of being pressed down, weighed down, or burdened, which affects a person physically, mentally, spiritually, and relationally.*

In other words, depression is not a state of mind but a state of *being*.

Depression is not a state of mind but a state of being.

A Complex Yet Common Disorder

Depression is a common disorder and a major cause of disability worldwide. According to the two largest and best-designed studies performed in the United States in recent years, the prevalence of depression serious enough to warrant treatment ("major" or "clinical" depression[1]) is between 5 and 10 percent,[2] although only 1 to 3 percent of Americans receive treatment for depression in any given year.[3] This means that between 14 million and 28 million Americans are suffering from depression as you read this. Women are more likely than men to experience depression by a ratio of about three to one. According to the American Psychiatric Association, 5 to 12 percent of women and 2 to 3 percent of men meet the criteria for major depression.[4]

It is possible that this discrepancy is related to the fact that, while women often talk about their problems and verbalize their feelings, men typically suffer in silence, immerse themselves in their work as a distraction from their pain, and dull that pain with drugs or drown it in alcohol (men have at least twice the rate of alcoholism as women).[5] Some men would prefer to develop more socially acceptable stress-related illnesses, such as heart disease or ulcers, than to have it known that they are consulting a professional for depression. Other masks of masculine melancholy include difficulty forming intimate relationships, abusive behavior, and rage.

The World Health Organization predicts that by 2020 depression will be the second-leading cause of disability in the world, second only to heart disease.

In the year 2000, according to the World Health Organization's project *The Global Burden of Disease,* major depression was the fourth-leading cause of disability in the world overall and the second-leading cause of disability for persons aged fifteen to forty-four. The same study predicted that by 2020 depression would be the second-leading cause of disability in the world, second only to heart disease.[6] *Disability,* as used here, means impairment of normal human abilities in such arenas as maintaining relationships with family or friends, fulfilling one's job responsibilities, or being able to relax and enjoy such things as recreation or vacations. Lifetime occurrence of depression is estimated at between 10 and 25 percent for women and between 5 and 12 percent for men.[7]

Major depression is marked by the presence, intensity, and longevity of a significant number of symptoms known to be associated with this disorder, including (but not limited to) depressed mood, loss of interest or pleasure, feelings of guilt or low self-worth, disturbed sleep or appetite, low energy, and poor concentration.[8] It is a complex disorder that affects the whole person, regardless of its causes, which is why the most effective treatment usually involves some form of counseling as well as medical intervention, pursued as early as possible after a diagnosis has been made.

The longer depression goes untreated, the harder it will be to treat effectively. Thankfully, we live in an era in which the downward spiral of depression can often be reversed through the cooperative effort of well-informed experts willing to confront what author Andrew Solomon called "the noonday demon"[9] with an arsenal of medical, psychological, sociological, and spiritual treatments. Such a multifaceted process can facilitate the release of a depressed person from what has seemed like an inescapable dank, dark dungeon—one that depressed people only a generation ago often endured in agonized silence.

As persons who have benefited ourselves from some of these treatments, we see them as gifts from God that cannot in good conscience be withheld from those who need them on any basis—theological, philosophical, theoretical, or otherwise. We'll have a lot more to say about this in chapter 9 on treating depression with antidepressant medication.

Classifying depression according to its causes (the fancy word is *etiology*) is not as helpful as was once thought because depression comes with many faces, all of them sad and streaked with tears. However, classifying a patient's depression by its apparent primary cause can aid those who are trying to formulate and implement an effective treatment plan.

Basic Types of Depression

There are four basic types of depression: situational depression, developmental depression, spiritual depression, and biological depression—all of them with some level of negative relational ramifications. For the sake of treatment and collaboration among providers of treatment, most depressions can fit into these categories. However, it is crucial for patients, their loved ones, and the professionals treating them to remember that types of depression tend to overlap with one another. Rarely does a person develop depression from a single underlying cause. Thus, in a very real sense, each person's depression is unique to him or her.

For example—Sarah's depression (cited earlier) was primarily *situational,* though over time it developed biological and some spiritual components. By comparison, one of our colleagues, psychiatrist Dr. Stephen Mory, experienced a depression with *developmental* roots but which also had biological and spiritual components. This is his story.

"My mother had a tendency toward depression, and I think I learned this method of dealing with stress, including anxiety, fear, and loss, from her. The lessons began early. She had experienced placenta abruptio (a condition in which the placenta starts to separate from the uterus) prior to my birth. She was in bed alone at home, terrified, and going into shock when my father found her and rushed her to the hospital.

"I believe that even as an infant I internalized her tendency toward depression," Dr. Mory wrote. "I received her emotions of fear and hopelessness by mutual experience.

"The first clinical depression I recognized in myself was about a year of depressed mood, frequent crying, and feeling helpless and inadequate that happened at age ten, when my oldest brother died in the Air Force. My parents were both devastated by grief, but my mother went into a severe depressive episode for two or three years. I remember that whenever she cried, I cried for her and for me. This was the trigger for my first depression, which eventually resolved on its own. There were some shorter depressive episodes in my adolescence and again in medical school."

We'll return to Dr. Mory's story in chapter 11, on the role of family and friends, to see how love helped overcome and reverse the negatives of his childhood, which may have given rise to his depression later in life. At age ten he not only lost his brother, but he also lost his parents emotionally for a while to their grief, eventually taking his mother's pain

There are four basic types of depressive disorders: situational depression, developmental depression, biological depression, and spiritual depression. These commonly overlap each other. Therefore, each person's depression is unique to him or her.

Spiritual depression is an uncommon diagnosis, at least in most medical settings, but we believe that depression can both originate with spiritual causes and have spiritual effects.

inside and becoming her burden-bearer. Childhood deprivation of this nature often produces the impression of carrying a heavy weight through life—this feeling is called "depression."

Spiritual depression is an uncommon diagnosis, at least in most medical settings, but we believe that depression can originate with spiritual causes and can have spiritual effects. As with the other types of depression, spiritual depression can have situational, biological, and even developmental components, but spiritual depression is the primary classification when the main issues are those for which faith, reconciliation with God, and the experience of his grace and forgiveness are the most effective treatments.

For example, I (DB) lost my three-year-old son, Jonathan, to a rare illness in 1978. This loss (a situation) launched me into an extended struggle with guilt and other spiritual factors, resulting in long-term biochemical depletion and relational disintegration within my family. Through the lens of twenty-five years of struggling with depression, I now see the spiritual components as primary, since it was my disappointment, even anger, with God for allowing such a loss to occur that fueled the sense of guilt that nearly drove me mad. Here is a condensed account of what happened, including how the God with whom I strove and from whom I was alienated for years remained gracious enough to forgive.

"After the Mayo Clinic's autopsy report suggested that dehydration contributed to the brain damage that had led to Jonathan's death, I became the accused, jury, and judge in a downwardly spiraling guilt trip that led me into obsessions and compulsions that took years to eliminate. I held myself responsible for Jonathan's death because, in the early morning hours before his illness manifested itself, I had told him not to take a drink after he'd thrown up yet another time. Of course, this was because I didn't want him to become nauseated again.

"Everyone tried to convince me that it wasn't my fault. But it didn't matter what anyone said—in other words, the difference between true and false guilt was irrelevant to me as it is to most depressed people. The whole thing was a matter of the heart, and a heart that has turned away from God, while at the same time yearning for his comfort, is a sitting duck for all kinds of spiritual and psychological anomalies.[10]

"In 1996, having carried the weight of this guilt for almost two decades, I was privileged to spend some time bow hunting for elk in Wyoming's Bighorn Mountains. One day during that hunt, I returned to the same meadow where shortly following Jonathan's death I had sat and tried to make some sense of all that had just taken place. This time I sat in about the same spot looking out over the same mountains, still asking some of the same questions, and still to some degree suffering under my self-imposed sentence of lifelong unhappiness, which was what I thought I deserved for failing my son.

"As I sat there meditating on these things, I realized there were still some issues between God and me, one of which was that I had never thanked God in the context of what had happened, as the apostle Paul admonishes: 'In everything give thanks; for this is God's will for you in Christ Jesus' (1 Thess. 5:18 NASB). By this I mean that I had not thanked God for being with me through it all and especially for never turning from me even during times when I turned from him. So in a simple prayer I said, 'Thank you, Lord. Thank you.'

"Nothing really dramatic happened in that moment—no flash of light, no trumpet blast—but when I turned around, behind me in the meadow, where there had been no animals when I sat down, stood a domestic sheep. I had no idea where it had come from, but it was certainly out of place because a lone sheep in that wilderness would likely become lunch in short order for a mountain lion or bear.

"As I looked at the sheep through my binoculars, it turned and looked at me. Its face seemed worn and its wool ancient and shaggy. Suddenly I realized that whatever was happening had been orchestrated by God, who was at that moment saying: 'Behold, the Lamb of God who takes away the sin of the world!' (John 1:29 NASB).

"As a writer, I dwell in the land of symbols (for that is what words are). So the Lord knew that the best way to reach past my troubled mind to my bleeding heart to purge the vestiges of my obsessive guilt and open the way for reconciliation with him was through a symbol as powerful as this one. In other words, he met me where I was in order to take me where he wanted me to go."

Biological depression is the fourth type of depression. This is the area in which many physicians and psychotherapists focus their primary attention, which may not be in their patient's best interest. While the most common pathway of depression is biochemical depletion, treating only this aspect of the disorder does not ordinarily bring long-term resolution because it is only one factor in a constellation of causes. By *common pathway* we mean that most people with clinical depression are experiencing biochemical depletion to one degree or another, either as a primary cause or as a result of situational, developmental, or spiritual factors.

Although the most common pathway of depression is biochemical depletion, treating only this aspect of the disorder ordinarily will not bring long-term resolution because it is only one factor in a constellation of causes.

Depression that is primarily biological is particularly insidious because it may seem to appear out of nowhere. Quite often this Hydra (a many-headed mythological creature that grew two more heads for each one that was cut off) first rears its ugly head during late childhood or early adolescence.

Traci was eleven years old, in fifth grade, when she started having uncontrollable crying spells right in the middle of school for no apparent reason except a deep sadness she couldn't explain. She was mortified and ashamed, thinking something was wrong with her, but all she could do was put her head down on her desk and sob.

During her teen years Traci suffered horribly with the normal ups and downs of being a teenager as well as with her secret deep sadness and misery. She was consumed with shame and haunted by the fear that she couldn't feel normal and seemed to have no control over her low moods. By age fifteen these feelings had converted to self-loathing, which led to her first serious thoughts of suicide. She became a Christian that year, which probably saved her life.

Traci's newfound faith brought exhilaration and hope, but within a few years her depression (though she did not know that was the source of her suffering) had dragged her lower than before. She remained highly functional through her twenties—an overachiever whose writing and creativity were driven by the power of private pain and whose focus on performance was driven by the need to avoid feeling the full weight of that pain.

In the summer of 1993, however, the pressure and pretending caught up with Traci. She'd had ample Christian counseling by that time without much effect. So one day she packed up her work and left it with her boss, informing him that she needed a leave of absence or she might come unglued. She didn't have a clue what was really wrong; she just assumed she was defective and hopeless and so wounded from childhood events that she would never be happy, though she deeply longed to know real joy.

Looking back now, Traci can see that she should have been hospitalized in 1993, but in her usual fashion she "gutted it out," mostly hiding in her house for several weeks. She tried a trip to the ocean—previously her favorite place in the world, but this time all she wanted to do was walk in and drown. On her flight home, Traci paged through a travel magazine. There she discovered a magazine article by Colette Dowling excerpting her book, *You Mean I Don't Have to Feel This Way?* For the first time Traci realized that what was wrong with her had a name: clinical depression. Hugely relieved and frightened, she sought psychiatric help soon after her return home, as a result of which her major depressive disorder was finally diagnosed and treatment with antidepressant medication initiated.

Prior to this, Traci acknowledges, no amount of counseling or activities associated with her faith had been at all effective in her battle against depression. From the vantage point of her remission from depression, the most important lesson she has learned thus far is that for the rest of her life she will need to closely monitor her physical and mental health, because she simply cannot afford to ignore or avoid early symptoms or triggers.

"Having this disorder caused me both great shame and great anger for many years," Traci said, "but now I am just exceedingly grateful that there is help for me. I have learned that I can live a normal and happy life as long as I am careful to stay healthy and make use of any and all therapies that work for me. I've also learned that I am completely powerless over this disorder and that my symptoms have nothing to do with my character, my circumstances, my attitude, or even my faith, so simply trying harder to solve my problems in isolation is a waste of time and can be self-abusive."

In terms of advice to her fellow sufferers, Traci said, "Don't be afraid to go to any length necessary in order to find relief. Educate yourself and take personal responsibility for your health. Finally, avoid if you can or at least ignore people who are ignorant, whether by chance or by choice, about the complex nature of depression. Your burden is great enough without allowing them to add to it."

Most people with clinical depression are experiencing biochemical depletion to one degree or another.

Toward Hope

In this introduction we have tried to provide an overview of depression, from the definitions we're using to examples of all four primary types of this disorder: situational, developmental, spiritual, and biological. While the primary types of depression tend to overlap and a person with depression can experience multiple causes simultaneously, using such designations can still be valuable in providing a starting point for understanding and treating depression.

Most likely, if you're a person with depression, you have identified with one or more (perhaps many) of the symptoms described in the cases you've just read. If so, it is crucial that you realize that this does not mean that you are "mentally ill" (a term that is stigmatizing, in our opinion) but that *you are human*, as are all the people who have shared their stories. The reason they've chosen to be so transparent with such personal information is because they want you to know (especially if you are a person with depression) that you, like them, can function well, even as you and your loved ones learn to live with this disorder in a positive and productive way.

All of the cases cited describe people who are professionals with excellent credentials and impressive resumes. Knowing this should increase your hope that you too can emerge from the darkness that may seem impenetrable much of the time. We wish to inspire your family, friends, and other caregivers with this same hope.

One of our goals as we have created this book is that you would embrace hope (and be embraced by it and its Source). The fact is that nobody this side of heaven is perfect—whether we're speaking in the context of depression or anything else. As we see it, the main issue for believers who wish to learn to live with and, if possible, move beyond depression is not *being* but *becoming*—specifically, becoming all we can become in Christ. Part of this process of growth is learning to use our difficulties as an opportunity for witness to the fact that God exists and that he is willing to entrust his message of reconciliation and wholeness to earthen vessels like us.

Questions for Reflection

1. Identify points where your experience is similar to one or more of the cases in this chapter.

2. Does knowing that others have experienced (and more than survived) struggles like yours give you hope? If so, try to express this hope in a sentence and record it in your journal (see below).

3. Why do you think Christians tend to hide from others the full depths of their depression when they are in the midst of the struggle (or even afterward)?

4. If living with depression is like a long journey for which you may need companions and/or guides, what kind of credentials or characteristics would you wish them to have?

5. What analogies come to mind for depression? Example: It is like trying to swim in mud.

6. If you are struggling with depression (or living with/caring for someone who is), based on this chapter can you identify whether the depression is primarily developmental, situational, biological, or spiritual?

7. We suggest that you begin a journal if you don't already have one. A journal can be a notebook of any kind in which you record your thoughts, insights, questions, hopes, fears, prayers, and so forth over a period of time. One value of keeping a journal is that it can provide, retrospectively, a vivid reminder of how you were doing during certain periods of your life.

   Here's a suggestion for how to use your journal: Read Psalm 42 (Psalm 43 is its reprise), which describes what sounds like depression; for example, "My soul thirsts for God. . . . My tears have been my food day and night" (vv. 2–3). Yet these psalms also include some self-counseling: "I remember as I pour out my soul: how I used to go with the multitude, leading the procession to the house of God, with shouts of joy and thanksgiving among the festive throng. Why are you downcast, O my soul? Why so disturbed within me? Put your hope in God, for I will yet praise him, my Savior and my God" (vv. 4–5).

   In your journal write today's date. Then think of one thing for which you can praise God at this moment. (It can be the simplest thing, like the memory of a way he has blessed you recently or in the past.) Pause and express this to God in a very simple prayer, such as: "Dear God, thank you for . . ." and then write down that prayer.

   Finally, ask yourself: How might praising God even when I feel like I'm stuck in the muck of despair be one pathway toward joy again? Don't forget to write your answer in your journal.

Personal Wholeness Self-Check

Instructions: These statements and the Wheel of Wholeness that follows may help you establish a baseline in terms of your current health in a broad sense. Completing this now will give you a way to evaluate your progress as a result of reading this book (and possibly participating in a discussion group).

Wholeness is a dynamic sense of overall well-being—physically, emotionally, spiritually, and relationally—that affects a believer's ability to exhibit qualities consistent with knowing Jesus Christ as Savior and Lord. This definition reflects one of the Bible's key passages describing dynamic faith (see 2 Peter 1:3–11) in which the apostle Peter says that if the qualities of faith, goodness, knowledge, self-control, perseverance, godliness, brotherly kindness, and love are yours in increasing measure, your knowledge of Jesus Christ will be both effective and productive.

Part 1

Estimate your *present* position by giving yourself a score on a scale of 0 to 10 in each area. Respond to the statement for each as best you can. Note: There are no right and wrong responses, only *your* responses. (0 = Not at all true of me; 10 = Very true of me)

1. Mind: I have peace of mind.

    0   1   2   3   4   5   6   7   8   9   10

2. Emotions: I am emotionally healthy.

    0   1   2   3   4   5   6   7   8   9   10

3. Peace with Self: I have a healthy level of self-respect.

    0   1   2   3   4   5   6   7   8   9   10

4. Body: I take care of myself physically, doing what I can to maintain my health.

    0   1   2   3   4   5   6   7   8   9   10

5. Home Relationships: My relationships at home reflect security and love.

    0   1   2   3   4   5   6   7   8   9   10

6. Friendships: My friendships outside my home are mutually beneficial.

    0   1   2   3   4   5   6   7   8   9   10

7. Church: My relationships with people in my church are positive and constructive.

    0   1   2   3   4   5   6   7   8   9   10

8. World: I want my life experiences (positive and negative) to help others in some way.

    0   1   2   3   4   5   6   7   8   9   10

9. Will: My decisions are consistent with my understanding of the will of God.

    0   1   2   3   4   5   6   7   8   9   10

10. Spiritual Maturity: I believe that I am spiritually mature.

    0   1   2   3   4   5   6   7   8   9   10

11. Loving God: My love for God is deep and strong.

    0   1   2   3   4   5   6   7   8   9   10

12. Loved by God: I feel secure (accepted and affirmed) when I think of God's love for me.

    0   1   2   3   4   5   6   7   8   9   10

13. Knowing God: I know God in a personal sense.

    0   1   2   3   4   5   6   7   8   9   10

Your score:

Add your individual scores together. The total can serve as an indicator of your sense of personal wholeness at this time. The divisions below are not based on scientific evidence but on doctoral studies of the tool's author with the help of several friends.

For example, if your total score is:

34 or less: there is room for growth, and we hope this book will help you;

35–64: you may be struggling in some areas, but you are growing;

65–88: your sense of wholeness is probably about average, yet there's still room for growth;

89–117: you feel that you are well adjusted, overall, while also still in process;

118 and up: you haven't left much room for growth, but perhaps as a result of reading this book you'll discover one or two things that could be improved.

Part 2

Using the categories/arenas of life in Part 1, list the three areas in which you think you need the most improvement.

1. _____

2. _____

3. _____

Part 3

To visualize your initial responses in Part 1, record them with an X on the Wheel of Wholeness below. Note: 0 is at the center; 10 is at the circumference.

Part 4

Review your responses to the statements in Part 1, placing an O (like a target) on the line under each category to indicate where you would like to be three months from now. Place the O's on the appropriate spokes of the Wheel of Wholeness to indicate your current goals in each area.

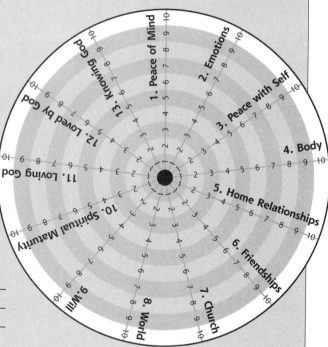

CHAPTER 2

Depression Is a Whole-Person Disorder

At nineteen I quit college and then lost my full-time job," Mary said about her first episode of depression. "I was unable to look for another job, living at home, dependent on my parents. None of us realized I had depression that could be treated. No one knew how to help or deal with me. I felt very alone.

"I continued attending church but withdrew from everything else and lost most of my friends. Most mornings I couldn't get out of bed. I felt guilty and lazy about my inability to get a job and function in a normal way. I got to the point where the only thing I could believe was that God existed. His personal love and care for me did not seem possible. I continued in this state for years, until it finally resolved by itself. I got a job, made some friends, found an apartment, and started living a normal life again.

"When my second depressive episode descended upon me at age thirty-three, I was working, supporting myself, and actively involved in a church. This time I knew I had depression. I went to an internist complaining that I was depressed and also tired all the time. His exam revealed a racing heart and severe high blood pressure. His goal became to treat my high blood pressure to reduce the danger of a stroke and/or heart attack. The process of finding the right drug and dosage for this took more than a year.

"It was only after several office visits and my persistence that the internist understood that I was clinically depressed. He kept thinking I would feel better when my blood pressure and heart rate problems were solved. He finally prescribed medication for the depression.

"I continued to be depressed, so the dosage was increased. I had an evaluation with a psychiatrist who recommended talk therapy and another increase in the dose of the antidepressant. After following this regimen for over a year I eventually felt better. Gradually, we were able to reduce my medications and finally eliminate them.

"During this time two of my good friends at church had moved out of the state, and I withdrew from the Bible study I was involved in due to my extreme fatigue. I did not have anyone to turn to who had the spiritual maturity to deal with my severe needs. So I sought ministry from my pastor and the elders at my church. I met with them as a group and shared my health problems. They prayed for me, but they would not make a plan for follow up. I was told, 'We will be in touch.' They did nothing else to assist me. After three weeks, I had a conversation of less than two minutes with an elder after church. A week later, I called the pastor, stating my continuing need for ministry. We spoke briefly, and I was assured that someone would call me back in two weeks to see how I was doing. That did not occur. It was three weeks before I spoke to the pastor again, and he could not seem to understand that I was ill and needed to know that the leadership of the church (and God) cared about me. After several more attempts to communicate with my newly assigned elder, I sent a letter to the elders stating my continuing need for ministry and my disappointment at their inability to minister to me.

"This culminated in a very distressing meeting with the pastor in which he acknowledged that the church had failed to minister to me during my illness, partly because they did not understand the seriousness of my condition. He then told me that it was my responsibility to forgive them, but that they would not try to find a way to meet my needs or minister to me. I could not believe I was hearing this. (I had taken someone with me to this meeting, and he could not believe this either.) I told the pastor that there was no reason for me to continue going to his church. I did not return to the church and never saw that pastor again.

"Four months passed before I received a letter from the church elders apologizing for their failure to minister to me and offering to try to find a way to meet my needs. By that time I was attending another church.

"My family recommended that I contact another pastor. He willingly met with me periodically to encourage me and to help me deal with my various life issues. He understood that I was ill and was eager to help me see that I did not have to face my illness alone. He ministered to me with the care and concern I had been requesting from my previous church. I starting attending and later joined his church.

"Although it was difficult, I also reached out and asked an acquaintance if she would meet with me regularly to talk and pray. She agreed to do this and helped me keep the faith and cling to the hope that I would return to health. Her love and prayers for me helped me get through this difficult time, preventing me from completely losing my relationship with the Lord.

"When I was forty-two, I had my third episode of depression. I recognized the symptoms, and my internist immediately prescribed the medication I had taken in the past. This time the medication did not help, so we tried several different medications and dosages. I remained severely depressed, so the internist finally referred me to a psychiatrist, who prescribed still more medications and dosages. I also resumed talk therapy as well. Since I was having suicidal thoughts daily, the psychiatrist put me in a day hospital program. I went to the hospital from 9:00 A.M. until 3:00 P.M. daily for two weeks. I participated in education, group therapy, goal-setting sessions, occupational therapy, and consultations with the medical team. After we made major changes to the medications and I was improving, I was released from the program.

"The goal of some of my previous doctors had been to eventually get me off my medications, but after hearing my history, the psychiatrist treating me now said I should be on medication the rest of my life. He explained that the right medications would help control my depression, but they could not cure it. His goal is to help me return to 'at my best' instead of 'not currently depressed.' We stay in contact at three-month intervals.

"Spiritually, although I've continued attending church (not always consistently), sometimes it has been hard to feel loved by God when life has been so difficult. Thankfully, a special friend has helped me through these dark times, sticking with me to show that, indeed, someone really does care.

"As I look back on more than twenty-five years of living with depression, one remarkable thing is that even when I was extremely ill, with much effort, I could smile and laugh and carry on a normal conversation. Many people I had daily contact with were unaware of my illness. No one at my current job knows I have this illness, although several friends, my immediate family, and some of my extended family know what I've been through. Very few people know I was in a hospital program, because I still feel that I need to hide my history, afraid that I will be misunderstood or lose my job. Most people know I have high blood pressure and diabetes and take medications and insulin injections daily, but I have kept my depression hidden. I weigh carefully what I reveal to others, even friends."

Mary's depression is most likely primarily biological with psychological, situational, and spiritual components and also with a significant social impact. Many depressed people like Mary expend lots of energy hiding their illness in one way or another, which drains their emotional reserves. This makes it more difficult for loved ones to understand them and for providers of professional care to properly diagnose and treat the depression itself rather than just its symptoms.

Depression, a Continuum of Pain

Depression affects people like Mary, Traci, Sarah, Dave, Steve, and a multitude of others who, for one reason or another, at one time or another, to one degree or another, feel pressed down by life. While individual reactions may vary even to the same event (for example, the reactions of spouses to a common loss) and the degree of the resulting depression may also vary, most depressive experiences and their symptoms lie along a seemingly interminable continuum of pain. This is one reason why the disorder is more difficult to recognize, diagnose, and treat than a disease like diabetes, for example. Yet this continuum of pain and symptoms also is a source of hope to those of us who have shared this pathway, because whether our depression is mild or severe, it's encouraging to know that someone else understands.

Depression is powerful. It may seem to well up from the chest or heart region. It is characterized by feelings of sadness, loss of interest, lack of motivation, and other symptoms described already through the cases you've read and which are discussed more fully later in this chapter. Everyday events are seen in a negative light, and positive experiences and circumstances are discounted or ignored.

Mild depression may commence after an argument with a loved one, a bad day at the office, or a loss or disappointment of almost any kind. Sometimes this negative mood is called "the blues." Usually it doesn't last long.

On the other hand, there is another *creature* with the same last name—"depression"—but whose first name is "major" (or "clinical"). With this creature, or perhaps *monster,* depressive feelings deepen and last for days, months, even years. They begin to overwhelm a person so that he or she can no longer function at work or within the family. There's no energy or desire to do anything, and the person may withdraw in order to avoid having to fulfill even the smallest request or expectation, as he or she feels there is nothing more to give.

Biochemistry and Depression

Some people have biochemical problems with their pancreas. This results in diabetes. Others have problems with their lungs. This may take the form of cystic fibrosis or asthma. Still others develop problems with their joints such as rheumatoid arthritis, with their muscles and nerves such as polio or muscular dystrophy, with the heart such as rheumatic fever, or with the thyroid gland such as hypothyroidism (which itself can be a biological cause of depression). All biological diseases have biochemical components. For every organ in the body there is an illness that affects the functioning of that organ.

Since the brain is a physical organ, we should expect there to be illnesses that affect its ability to function. Alzheimer's disease is an example of a medical illness that affects the surface areas of the brain and parts of the brain that control memory. Parkinson's disease is another example of a disease that affects the part of the brain called the *substantia nigra,* impairing a person's physical functioning, causing him or her to shake and move more slowly and stiffly. Inherited predispositions to both Alzheimer's disease and Parkinson's disease increase the likelihood that a person will develop these conditions at some point.

Similarly, when people inherit a tendency to develop high blood pressure, they may be more likely to experience a stroke. If that stroke happens to occur in the frontal lobes of the brain, then the affected person will experience what is called "disinhibition." In other words, their will may become paralyzed so they can no longer inhibit or stop socially unacceptable behaviors. A formerly proper and gracious older woman may suddenly become sexually uninhibited or may start cursing and swearing, even if this never occurred before.

Another area of the brain is called the limbic system. The limbic system is the center of emotion. From it arise expressions of anger, rage, feeding behavior, sleep, sexual behaviors, and other basic human instincts. Together with the temporal lobes (which are located nearby), the limbic system also enables us to experience feelings of joy, happiness, wonder, and awe. Illnesses exist that affect this part of the brain. One of them is called depression. With depression, key cells both in the limbic system and other areas throughout the brain become less able to produce chemicals such as serotonin, norepinephrine, and dopamine. These chemicals are called biogenic amines (or neurotransmitters). They are responsible for maintaining a positive mood and optimistic outlook.

Most depressive experiences and their symptoms lie along a seemingly interminable continuum of pain.

The most effective treatment for depression is a cooperative, multidisciplinary effort that considers all arenas of the depressed person's life.

The biological symptoms of depression have been documented by careful scientific research that has been replicated by many research groups in the United States and around the world. Levels of neurotransmitters can be measured in the fluid surrounding the brain and spinal cord of people who are depressed or have attempted or committed suicide.[1]

When the normal level of these neurotransmitters in the brain becomes altered or depleted as a result of situational, developmental, or spiritual stressors (causes), the person may experience loss of interest or feelings of guilt, worthlessness, self-condemnation, sadness, or failure—in other words, depression. In such cases, the biochemical depletion may be more a result of than the cause of the depression. In biological depression, by contrast, a biochemical imbalance may be the disorder's primary cause. In any case, the common pathway of all major depression is biochemical. This is why the common denominator of all treatment for major depression—whatever its primary cause—should be medical in nature. We'll return to this later.

Causes of Depressive Disorder

Major depression (see the symptoms later in this chapter) is called a "disorder," which meshes very well with our definitions of both depression and wholeness since the person's state of existence is disordered and he or she most likely feels fragmented to some degree. Depressive disorder can come on after a severe loss or multiple losses and, therefore, can be linked to circumstances. It may be tied to unmet emotional needs while growing up, it may have spiritual roots, or it may be primarily a biological illness that is genetically inherited. Most often these causes overlap, as we said in the previous chapter. Before describing each type of depression, we want to emphasize that the most effective treatment for depression, regardless of its cause (or overlapping causes) is a cooperative, multidisciplinary effort that considers all arenas of the depressed person's life—emotional, relational, spiritual, and physical.

Situational Depression

This kind of depression comes on after a person has undergone a severe stress. Situational stressors can be negative or apparently positive experiences, such as moving, taking a new job, and so forth. Depending upon a person's vulnerability (including developmental and biological predispositions) more or less stress can precipitate a situational depression, though no two people react identically, even to the same stressor.

All of us have a certain vulnerability to depression. Given the *right kind* of stress, the *right magnitude* of stress, and the *right duration* of stress, it is possible, perhaps even normal, for *anyone* to become depressed to some degree.

Sometimes a person may feel pressed down by the results of poor decisions or actions. For example, cheating on one's income tax can land a person in jail. Cheating on one's spouse may result in a divorce or other family turmoil. Harboring resentments may generate internal stress that leads to depression. Sometimes one's response to difficulties (for example, being hit and injured by a drunk driver) can generate stress that in turn produces depression, as when the injured person turns to drugs or other substances in order to cope with the physical pain of the injury itself or related psychic pain. Such a pattern can even lead beyond depression to addiction, broken marriage, and the loss of one's job.

"Adjustment disorder" is the official psychiatric name for a situational depression that is relatively mild, occurring within three to six months of a stressful psychological or interpersonal event, that does not fulfill the criteria for major depression. An adjustment disorder, even if it is not classified as clinical depression, may cause significant impairment of social or occupational functioning. The most effective treatment is usually provided by a combination of professionals, including those who can prescribe and monitor response to antidepressant medication and those who provide psychotherapy (counseling) support. Counseling itself may come from more than one source in order to focus on specific needs, whether psychological, spiritual, or sociological.[2]

Given the right kind, *the* right magnitude, *and the* right duration *of stress, it is possible for* anyone *to become depressed to some degree.*

Developmental Depression

This form of depression is often chronic, lasting for years or, in some cases, for decades. It is sometimes called "characterological" (personality-related) depression. Symptoms include a persistent inability to appreciate the positive aspects of life along with an almost obsessive preoccupation with the negative. By comparison with situational depression, current stressors in the depressed person's life, though they may intensify a developmental depression, are less important as a primary cause. Also less common is a strong genetic link, though there may be some family history of depression.

The dominant factor in developmental depression appears to be the experience of major losses during childhood or early deprivation of emotional needs. This does not necessarily imply that early care providers were abusive or neglectful, but it may mean that the needs of the child

The dominant factor in developmental depression appears to be the experience of major losses during childhood or early deprivation of emotional needs.

were so great that the care providers could not adequately meet them. For example, an emotionally needy infant may require almost constant attention at a time when a mother may be herself experiencing depression (as occurs for many women after childbirth). Similarly, marital or job stress or other significant stressors may distract parents away from the child during a critical developmental period.

Regardless of the circumstances, the way to wholeness for a person with developmental depression is not through blaming or bitterness but rather through forgiveness, the release of long-held grudges, and learning new patterns of relating to others through the help of a counselor or counselors. This psychotherapy is most effective when it is combined with treatment with antidepressant medication, which can remedy biochemical depletion in the person's brain that might otherwise hinder his or her ability to comprehend and respond to the counseling received.

Biological Depression

When underlying biological or genetic causes of depression are strong, it is called "biological depression." Often people inherit a form of depression from their parents that has been passed from generation to generation.

In February 2003, a report published in the *Wall Street Journal* announced that scientists at Myriad Genetics (Salt Lake City, Utah) had identified a gene that causes depression. This gene, named DEP1 (most likely for "depression gene 1") was isolated through the study of hundreds of Mormon families and their genealogical records.[3] Another study, published in the July 18, 2003 issue of *Science* magazine, examined why stressful experiences lead to depression in some people but not in others. Results indicated that adults who carried a short form of the gene 5-HTT (which helps regulate serotonin) were more prone to depression after serious life events than were adults who carried the long form of the same gene.[4] Although a lot more research lies ahead in this arena, these discoveries represent a giant leap forward in the science of depression.

For many years scientists have known by observation that certain forms of depression seemed to have some genetic basis, as they tended to run in families. All that is known for sure is that some individuals inherit a general vulnerability, since not everyone with a particular gene (or combination of genes) develops depression. This individual variation is most likely true of all inherited depressions, so one cannot use "being born that way" as an excuse for acting irresponsibly or refusing to pursue help if depression sets in. In a spiritual sense, this parallels the fact that although we are all born with (i.e., we inherit) an inclination to sin, God still holds us personally accountable when we give in to temptation.

Inherited depression is often more severe than other types of depression and less responsive to social support, psychotherapy, or spiritual forms of treatment. In persons biologically predisposed to depression—including the most devout believers—a small error in judgment, a slight indiscretion, or a minor interpersonal conflict may trigger a full-blown depressive episode.

When this happens to believers, no matter how much they pray, go to church, or read the Bible, they still suffer from depression. No matter how much they confess their sins, treat others kindly, or "lay down their lives for God," they still remain depressed. Standing in judgment of such persons only intensifies their pain, making matters worse for all concerned. However, encouragement, support, and assistance in pursuing every available avenue of treatment can help alleviate their pain.

In persons biologically predisposed to depression—including the most devout believers—a small error in judgment, a slight indiscretion, or a minor interpersonal conflict may trigger a full-blown depressive episode.

Spiritual Depression

Depression may be primarily spiritual in nature. In other words, for some people the causes of depression (which may include situational, developmental, or biochemical components) are rooted in the realm of the spirit.

Some become depressed due to feelings of guilt over their sins. Several of David's psalms, for example, seem linked to his infamous affair with Bathsheba and related events. He wrote, "When I kept silent, my bones wasted away through my groaning all day long. *For day and night your hand was heavy upon me;* my strength was sapped as in the heat of summer" (Ps. 32:3–4, emphasis added; see also Ps. 51). The italicized phrase clearly describes depression—feeling pressed down by life is one thing; being pressed down by the hand of God is another! The treatment for this expression of depression is confession, as David describes in the next sentence. The sooner this happens for a person depressed by guilt, the less intense his or her spiritual depression should become. The longer one's bones waste away through hiding sin, the deeper one's depression will become. Many spiritual counselors focus primarily on this arena. Some focus on it exclusively.

Depression related to guilt, however, can be two-faced. While true guilt may cause depression, depression may cause a person to feel truly guilty when there is no reason. Experientially, it makes little difference to the depressed person which type of guilt is fueling his or her depression, and this creates many rabbit trails for spiritual counselors who reject a cooperative, multidisciplinary approach.

While true guilt may cause depression, depression may cause a person to feel truly guilty when there is no reason.

There is more to spiritual depression than guilt; in other words, not all depression is related to sins, whether real or imaginary. (See chapter 4, "Ten Myths and Misconceptions," for more on this.) However, as with guilt, many of the following common elements in spiritual depression can be either causes or results, and it is not always easy to discern which came first.

Some may imagine that God doesn't love them, has deserted them, or is punishing them. Or they may feel that their faith community has turned its back on them. They may experience doubts about the reality or security of their faith. This kind of despair is fraught with uncertainty and a sense of hopelessness or helplessness.[5] Such feelings are extremely difficult for believers who formerly enjoyed a close personal relationship with God.

Henri Nouwen, one of our favorite writers on spiritual themes, described his own depression in these terms:

> Just when all those around me were assuring me they loved me, cared for me, appreciated me, yes, even admired me, I experienced myself as a useless, unloved, and despicable person. Just when people were putting their arms around me, I saw the endless depth of my human misery and felt that there was nothing worth living for. Just when I had found a home, I felt absolutely homeless. Just when I was being praised for my spiritual insights, I felt devoid of faith. Just when people were thanking me for bringing them closer to God, I felt that God had abandoned me. It was as if the house I had finally found had no floors. The anguish completely paralyzed me. I could no longer sleep. I cried uncontrollably for hours. I could not be reached by consoling words or arguments. I no longer had any interest in other people's problems. I lost all appetite for food and could not appreciate the beauty of music, art, or even nature. All had become darkness. Within me there was one long scream coming from a place I didn't know existed, a place full of demons.[6]

Similar musings of other spiritual guides through the ages suggest that depression of this type is not uncommon among those who are spiritually sensitive, especially when they view their own frailty in the light of God's perfection.[7] Those who strive to achieve a similar perfection as human beings often experience depression due to sense of failure caused by an inability to measure up to the impossibly high standards of perfectionism.

The most effective treatment for depressions arising from these sources is the application of grace to the places that hurt most. The apostle Paul described his own inner struggles in Romans 7:7–24, but note that he ended with these words of hope: "What a wretched man I am! Who will rescue me from this body of death? Thanks be to God—through Jesus Christ our Lord! . . . Therefore, there is now no condemnation for those who are in Christ Jesus" (Rom. 7:24–8:1). In Nouwen's case this grace was incarnated by several close friends who joined him on his unexpected journey to the point where he could once again hear the inner voice of love.

In his "cry of abandonment" while on the Cross, Jesus identified with the feeling of abandonment experienced by so many of his depressed brothers and sisters through the ages.

Several other common themes for believers experiencing depression include: shame, feeling that one's prayers are not being heard, or a pervasive sense of alienation or disconnection from the church and ultimately from God, as though he had deserted his own child. This is the perspective of Psalm 22:1–2, a psalm of David: "My God, my God, why have you forsaken me? Why are you so far from saving me, so far from the words of my groaning? O my God, I cry out by day, but you do not answer, by night, and am not silent."

Jesus adopted these words as his own when, as he took the sin of all mankind for all time on himself at the Cross, he experienced for at least that moment what so many believers through the ages have felt in one way or another—abandoned. Is it not possible that during that moment (as well as at other times) Jesus could identify with this aspect of depression, which so many of his brothers and sisters have experienced through the ages? Charles Spurgeon had no doubt about this. "It is a rule of the kingdom that all members must be like the head," Spurgeon said.

> But we must be like the head . . . in his humiliation, or else we cannot be like him in his glory. Now . . . our Lord and Savior Jesus Christ very often passed through much of trouble, without any heaviness . . . like a ship floating over the waves of the sea. But . . . at last the waves of swelling grief came into the vessel; at last the Savior himself, though full of patience, was obliged to say, "My soul is exceeding sorrowful, even unto death"; and [he] "began to be very heavy." What means that, but that his spirits began to sink! The Savior passed through the brook [of suffering], but he "drank of the brook by the way"; and we who pass through the brook of suffering must drink of it too. He had to bear the burden, not with his shoulders omnipotent, but with shoulders that were bending to the earth beneath the load. And you and I must not always expect a giant faith that can remove mountains. Sometimes even the grasshopper must be a burden, that we may in all things be like our head.[8]

Before leaving this topic, we want to note that unbelievers can also experience spiritual depression, in which case it may seem to them that

Often, after waking early, a depressed person cannot fall asleep again because regrets or worries beckon.

something is missing or that there is a void at the core of their being. The awareness of this inner emptiness can have a positive result, as it may help that person realize his or her need of God, who created humans with this God-shaped vacuum that only he can fill—with himself.

Resolution of spiritual depression is important whether or not people are believers, for when these struggles remain unresolved, a person's psychological and physical health may suffer. In a Duke University study, the mortality rate of those with unresolved spiritual issues was higher over two years of monitoring than persons without these struggles. The categories covered in this study were:

1. Wondered whether God had abandoned me;
2. Felt punished by God for my lack of devotion;
3. Wondered what I did for God to punish me;
4. Questioned God's love for me;
5. Wondered whether my church had abandoned me;
6. Decided the Devil made this happen;
7. Questioned the power of God.[9]

Depression (from mild to major) may arise from primarily spiritual issues. However, diagnosing and treating spiritual depression is complicated because it is difficult to know whether spiritual struggles are the primary cause of the depression or whether a depression from some other cause is making the person feel guilty, distant from God, or unloved by his or her faith community.

What Depression Looks Like

If a person is depressed, regardless of cause or severity, he or she will most likely exhibit some of the following patterns of thought or action. (Note: If the person exhibits several of these characteristics, he or she may be heading toward major depression, even if it has not been diagnosed yet. This should be ample reason for obtaining a professional evaluation.)

- *Difficulty in relationships.* In times of distress many people with depression tend to withdraw to the only apparently safe place—within themselves. Relationships, if they exist at all, are mostly superficial. Intimate relationships—knowing and being known—are threatening, sometimes because their low self-esteem warns that were they really known, they would not be liked anymore. This trait can also hinder one's relationship with God.

- *Irritability.* Some psychological schools of thought believe repressed anger to be the primary cause of depression. Our view is that when a person is depressed, anger may be a *cause* or it may be a *result* of the depression, and it is nearly impossible to tell which came first. In any case, anger is often present. It may rear its ugly head in a variety of ways, including fits of rage or outbursts over trivial matters. Such a pattern surely hinders one's ability to relate to anyone—whether spouse, family, friends, or God.

- *Problems sleeping.* This can go either way—depression is often accompanied by too little or too much sleep, typically too little. Depressed people have a lot on their minds. Often the processing of these concerns occurs late at night (hindering falling asleep) or early in the morning when, after waking, the person cannot fall asleep again because regrets or worries beckon. Either way, the result over time is physical exhaustion and biochemical depletion, since sleep is the body's normal way of maintaining, restoring, or renewing us. (Note: There are also medical causes of insomnia or hypersomnia—too much sleep—that may contribute to depression and should be evaluated by a physician.)

- *A broad search for causes and cures.* Depressed people are especially susceptible to suggestions from others regarding the causes and cures of their illness. From demon possession[10] as a cause to chiropractic adjustment as a cure, often they will consider just about anything to escape their anguish. Because they are running on empty most of the time due to the constant energy drain of depression, depressed people lack the emotional resources to resist suggestions they might ordinarily reject out of hand.

- *Fear of losing one's mind.* The pit of depression can be very deep. When it is at its worst and everything looks black, brown, or gray, a person may worry that he or she may go "over the edge" and hurt someone—including spouse, children, or self. In a sense, having a complete nervous breakdown can relieve some of the guilt that depressed people (especially depressed Christians) feel, since being able to give their rather nebulous constellation of symptoms a name other than depression might seem to legitimize their need for help.

Depressed people are especially susceptible to suggestions from others regarding the causes and cures of their illness.

A person's perception may be so warped by depression that he or she consistently adopts the most negative interpretation possible of present events or conversations.

- *A complex of new physical ailments.* Headaches, backaches, neck aches, joint pain, fatigue, TMJ (temporomandibular joint) syndrome, and gastrointestinal disorders are among the many physical symptoms that often accompany, and may disguise, depression. These symptoms are real; their pain is real. Yet until the depression itself is treated, the failure of physical symptoms to respond to medical treatment may mystify and frustrate both patient and physician.

- *Loss of energy.* Depressed people feel physically exhausted most of the time, perhaps because so much of their energy (psychic energy is still energy) is devoted to mulling over their problems. Completing routine tasks—paying bills, finishing yard work, doing the laundry, preparing a meal, cleaning the house, even taking care of matters relating to personal hygiene—can seem daunting.

- *Diminished libido (sexual drive).* Maintaining normal sexual relations with one's partner may seem impossible (and may be perceived as rejection by the other person).

- *Impaired memory and thinking.* Although memories of past failures remain (even if the perception of these may not be accurate), often a depressed person cannot remember events in the recent past or important matters in the present, such as appointments or other commitments, phone numbers, names of people, special events, and so forth. In addition, the person's perception may be so warped by depression that he or she consistently adopts the most negative interpretation possible of present events or conversations.

- *Change in eating patterns.* This, too, can go either way—eating too little or too much. In either case a perceptive observer will note a significant change in the person's weight over time. Also, lack of certain nutrients normally available through a healthy diet may contribute to depression in some people whose dietary practices are eccentric or significantly unbalanced.[11]

- *Feelings of worthlessness.* The guilt or shame felt by depressed people can be immeasurable. It is also usually beyond the reach of reason—as in, "But Dave, just think of how many people you've helped through the years." Or, "But Harold, Jesus took all our guilt and shame on himself at Calvary. Can't you just take yours to the Cross and leave it there?" These feelings of worthlessness, taken to an extreme, may tempt even a believer to consider ending his or her life, not only because the person believes that he or she does not deserve to live but also to put an end to the inconvenience and distress that his or her life causes others.

The guilt or shame felt by depressed people can be immeasurable and beyond the reach of reason.

How Major Depression Is Diagnosed

Depression arising from situational, developmental, biological, or spiritual causes can be mild and short-term or major (clinical) and possibly chronic (dysthymic). Persons who are mildly depressed may exhibit one or more of the following symptoms. Clinical depression is the diagnosis when at least five of the following nine symptoms of depression have been present for two weeks or longer and they are significantly interfering with functioning in social settings (including marriage and family relationships) or in the workplace:

- persistent sadness, unhappiness, or irritability
- lethargy or fatigue
- loss of interest in previously enjoyable activities
- sudden change in appetite
- disruption of normal sleep pattern
- feeling guilty or worthless
- moving about more slowly and sluggishly, or feeling restless and needing to move all of the time
- difficulty thinking or concentrating
- recurrent thoughts of suicide or death

Subtypes of Major Depression

A number of subtypes of major depression (called "course specifiers" in *DSM-IV*[12]) are worth knowing about. A course specifier describes special characteristics of a major depression related to its cause, presenting symptoms, or when it occurs. These specifiers distinguish one type of depression from other types and suggest what kind of treatment is likely to be effective. The most common subtypes are based on depression's severity, the presence of psychotic symptoms, the time of the year, or relationship to the birth of a child.

Severity. Major depression (at least five of the nine symptoms above) occurs on a continuum of severity, including mild, moderate, and severe.

One person may have only mild loss of interest in several different aspects of life whereas another person may have severe and profound loss of interest and inability to experience pleasure. A person can meet the criteria for diagnosis of major depression even when his or her symptoms are relatively mild. A person with moderate major depression may have more of these symptoms in a more severe form. A person with severe major depression will have most of the symptoms to a disrupting and paralyzing degree.

Psychosis. Psychotic depression is major depression accompanied by psychotic symptoms, including loss of contact with reality, paranoid delusions, or even hallucinations. These symptoms usually call for immediate hospitalization, since they are often severely disabling, disruptive relationally, and occasionally dangerous.

Correct diagnosis is very important in this case, since psychotic symptoms are also seen in several other psychiatric disorders. The depressed person may have an underlying bipolar disorder and be experiencing a mixture of depressive and psychotic symptoms or depression mixed with another psychotic disorder such as schizophrenia, in which case it is called schizoaffective disorder. Older adults, especially those with Alzheimer's disease or other dementia, are more likely than younger adults to have psychotic symptoms accompany their depression.

When psychotic depression occurs in older adults, electroconvulsive treatment (ECT) is particularly effective. (Note: We will return to this when we consider various treatments, but rest assured that today's ECT treatments are not like similar treatments you may have seen in movies. For example, in the 2002 movie *A Beautiful Mind,* the main character receives not ECT but insulin shock treatment, which causes a grand mal seizure in the patient.) Younger persons with depression and psychosis may be abusing hallucinogenic drugs, and this needs to be determined. In any case, when depression is accompanied by psychotic symptoms, antidepressants alone will not be enough. Antipsychotic medication or ECT must be given in addition to antidepressants for successful treatment.

Time of the year. Seasonal Affective Disorder (SAD) is a type of major depression whose cause seems linked to the amount of sunlight the person with this manifestation of depression receives on a daily basis. Typically, SAD appears at about the same time each year (usually in the winter). Its diagnosis is made when symptoms have appeared at the same time of year for at least two years in a row and the symptoms have resolved with the change of seasons. The most common symptoms are lethargy and irritability. There is no known cure for SAD, though it can be managed with medication, counseling, and light (photo) therapy—in which the patient is exposed to sunlight-emulating artificial lighting for a certain period daily as long as this therapy is needed.

Relationship to the birth of a child. Postpartum depression is a major depression that comes on after the birth of a child. Many women have a normal degree of postpartum blues following delivery that do not interfere with functioning. However, with the dramatic hormonal changes that occur in a woman's body after birth and the disruption of sleep and routine a newborn can introduce, a severe depression may develop that can endanger the life of the mother and the baby.

Bipolar Disorder

Bipolar disorder is a cyclic and recurrent mood disorder with a strong biological component. Without treatment (and even sometimes with treatment), a person with this disorder may experience depression for six to nine months and then experience a period of months or even years of complete wellness before another episode of depression comes on. Some people with bipolar disorder (which used to be called manic-depressive illness) experience cycles of mood that include periods of depression followed by a short period of normal mood and then by elevated mood characterized by euphoria, increased energy, decreased need for sleep, impatience, increased sexual interest, and great productivity (called mania or hypomania, depending on severity).

If at any time in life a depressed person has experienced an episode of mania that lasted for one week or longer, then that person is said to have bipolar disorder. When classic mania occurs (preventing the person from functioning at work or in relationships), it is called bipolar type I; if only hypomania occurs (milder symptoms that do not cause dysfunction), then it is called bipolar type II.

It is *extremely important* for a doctor to know if the depressed person has *ever* had a manic or hypomanic episode because this will significantly affect the treatment chosen. For example, if a person with bipolar disorder sees a doctor during an episode of depression and the doctor prescribes an antidepressant, this may throw the patient into a manic episode or may worsen the frequency of mood switches. Such a manic episode may be so disorganized and disruptive that the person may end up psychotic and in the hospital. For that reason, before treating this person's depression with an antidepressant, the doctor should first

It is extremely important for a doctor to know if the depressed person has ever had a manic or hypomanic episode because this will significantly affect the treatment chosen.

prescribe a mood stabilizer. If you have ever had mania or hypomania, always tell your doctor about this—whether or not the doctor remembers to ask about it.

All of the specifiers or types of major depression described earlier also apply to bipolar disorder, even though bipolar disorder is not considered a type of major depression. Thus, a person may have mild, moderate, or severe bipolar disorder. Bipolar disorder may or may not be accompanied by psychotic symptoms. An episode of depression or mania may recur at any time of year or at a particular time of the year (like SAD), or it may occur following the birth of a child.

Disease, Health, and Human Nature

Thus far in this book we have avoided as much as possible the use of the word *disease* to describe depression because it is defined in a variety of ways. For example, as recently as 1998 the U.S. Food and Drug Administration (FDA) tried to redefine the word *disease,* in part because the older definition (1993) was not inclusive enough to include conditions such as depression. The earlier definition said that disease involved "damage to an organ, part, structure, or system of the body such that it does not function properly (e.g., cardiovascular disease), or a state of health leading to such dysfunction (e.g., hypertension); except that diseases resulting from essential nutrient deficiencies (e.g., scurvy, pellagra) are not included in this definition."[13]

While most diseases either result in or are the result of measurable damage to an organ, part, structure, or system, it is not very easy to quantify this type of damage in relation to depression (and some other conditions, such as migraine). So in 1998 the FDA proposed the revised definition that disease is "any deviation from, impairment of, or interruption of the normal structure or function of any part, organ, or system (or combination thereof) of the body that is manifested by a characteristic set of one or more signs or symptoms, including laboratory or clinical measurements that are characteristic of a disease."[14]

Although this revision is more aligned with the root meaning of the word *disease* (*dis* = lack of/absence of + *ease* = comfort/freedom from care) and its normal meaning as used by doctors and patients, the FDA received more than 100,000 letters, most of them protesting the proposed change. (Many of these protests evidently came from individuals or groups whose products claimed to be able to prevent or reverse the "damage" referenced in the 1993 definition.) The redefinition of *disease* remains unresolved.

In order to define what we mean by the word *disease*, we would like to first consider the definition of the word *health*. This is easier, since in 1946 the World Health Organization adopted the following definition, which has not been amended since 1948: "Health is a state of complete physical, mental, and social well being and not merely the absence of disease or infirmity."[15]

It seems logical that if we accept this definition of health (adding the spiritual element), then disease is a state of existence in which a person experiences diminished physical, mental, spiritual, and social well-being. Since this definition of disease is consistent with our definition of depression, we can say that *depression is a disease that affects, to one degree or another, every arena of an affected person's state of existence.*

> *Depression is a disease that affects, to one degree or another, every arena of an affected person's state of existence.*

What Is Man?

The psalmist, David, who during his shepherding nights must have often gazed up at the stars, wondered aloud, "What is man that you are mindful of him, the son of man that you care for him?" (Ps. 8:4). Before we conclude this chapter, we'd like to ponder this question in relation to depression and its treatment, for one's view of human nature significantly influences how each person (whether patient, family, or professional provider) will proceed.

To start at the most basic level, it is obvious enough (though some would deny even this) that human beings are comprised of a physical or material entity called a "body" and a nonphysical (or immaterial) entity often called the "mind." In the Scriptures, this immaterial part is known by many names, including spirit, soul, heart, mind, inner man, inner person of the heart, and so forth. In fact, the King James version of the Old Testament uses twenty-eight different English words to translate the single Hebrew word *nephesh*, which ordinarily means "self" or "soul." The New Testament word translated "soul," "life," or "self," is *psuché*, from which we get the English word *psyche*, the verbal root of words such as *psychology, psychological*, and so forth. This word occurs more than a hundred times in the New Testament, for example in Matthew 10:28, where Jesus says, "Do not be afraid of those who kill the body but cannot kill the soul [*psuché*]."

Too often providers of care do not communicate well, if at all, with each other about a patient's needs, each treating the part that he or she knows best, perhaps convinced that healing in this arena will bring all the healing the patient needs.

Despite the wide variety of words used in the Bible to describe the immaterial part of human nature, the biblical view is that the material and immaterial aspects function as an essential unity until the material and immaterial are separated at death. Some Christians insist that this "unitary" perspective is the only acceptable biblical view, which is fine as far as it goes but not very helpful in discerning a patient's primary needs or designing a multidisciplinary treatment plan.

The most common secular construct of human nature is mind-body, while many secular models also include a social component. The result is that the most common model accepted in medicine or psychology is either two-part (biopsychological) or three-part (biopsychosocial).

Interestingly, a three-part construct of human nature is also a common model used by Christian counselors, pastors, and doctors today—the three elements being, however, body, soul, and spirit. Those who endorse this view often use 1 Thessalonians 5:23 as its basis: "May God himself, the God of peace, sanctify you through and through. May your whole spirit, soul and body be kept blameless at the coming of our Lord Jesus Christ." This model is useful as long as those who employ it do not forget that the divine perspective is that humans are single entities comprised of material and immaterial (or spiritual) components.

If a professional provider of care endorses the Christian three-part view, logic suggests that the patient's treatment can legitimately be divided among three providers of care. The pastor will deal with things of the spirit. The psychotherapist (counselor) will deal with matters of the mind, will, and emotions (what some call "the soul"). The physician will deal with physical symptoms. Too often, however, these individuals do not communicate well, if at all, with each other about a patient's needs, each treating the part that he or she knows best, perhaps convinced that healing in this arena will bring all the healing the patient needs.

For example, a member of the clergy may insist that a person's depression is entirely a spiritual matter. This minister is less likely to refer the patient in question for treatment of the body or soul. Psychotherapists sometimes adopt a similar mentality, insisting that if patients can resolve their emotional problems, learn new patterns of thought, and muster the will to follow through, they will recover. Physicians, even many Christian physicians, may perceive a patient's depression as primarily physical in nature, specifically, a biochemical imbalance for which modern medicine can provide assistance. Once the right medication at the right dose has been taken for a long enough period, the patient should be functioning normally again. In cases in which the main professional is a social worker, there will likely be a greater emphasis on the sociological factors of the patient's depression.

We believe it is in the depressed patient's best interests that a different standard of care be practiced that includes treatment of the body as well as the soul and/or spirit in every case, without neglecting the patient's social context. The primary implication of this standard of care is that, in order to ensure more complete and effective treatment of each patient with depression, all the professionals providing care must become better allies in the healing process. While it should not be left to the patient to request this alliance, making such a request would be entirely appropriate for a patient or loved one when it is obvious that the professional caregivers are not working as a team (or worse, are not interested in working as a team).[16]

Conclusion

We hope that this chapter has helped you gain insight, perhaps even a new perspective on depression as a whole-person disorder that is best treated by a cooperative, multidisciplinary team of providers of care. We trust that if you are depressed, you will neither resent nor resist the suggestion that true healing most likely will require treatment by more than one type of professional.

On the other hand, we hope you *will* resist any suggestion by *any* professional that his or her treatment is the only therapy you need. Difficult as it may be, since depression has most likely sapped most of your energy, you may need to become your own advocate for multispecialty treatment because you know this collaborative effort will provide the best context for your journey toward wholeness.

Finally, there is something we hope you won't do as a result of reading this chapter. We hope you won't permanently label yourself or someone you love who may be depressed. Doctors' diagnoses are not made in order to put people in boxes but to enable all interested parties, especially professionals, to discuss the situation and determine what treatment options might be most effective in a particular case. In most instances, clinical depression can be treated successfully. So rest assured, you will not always be "Dysthymia #102" or "Major Depression #657." You are a unique human being, not a diagnosis, and God loves you regardless of your diagnosis or the symptoms that may be pressing you

Depression is a whole-person disorder that is best treated by a cooperative, multi-disciplinary team of caregivers.

down at this moment. He desires the same thing you want—your victory in this battle so that when those who know you see your progress, they will demand to know the reason for the hope that is in you.

Questions for Reflection

1. If you could talk with Mary, the opening case in this chapter, what would you like to tell her?

2. If you could freeze-frame your advice to Mary and apply it to yourself, how might it sound? Write this advice to yourself in your journal.

3. Review the section "What Depression Looks Like." Which of these characteristics have you personally experienced or seen in others? Which of these do you think would be most difficult to resolve?

4. What are you going to say the next time anyone suggests that your depression (or the depression of someone you love) is purely spiritual and if you would just do this or that it would go away?

5. We referred to clinical depression as a "creature" or a "monster." If you agree with these descriptions, sketch this monster in your journal. If you want to be really creative, give it a name and describe in words or depict graphically what you would like to see happen to it.

6. If we all are, by God's design, inseparably composed of material and immaterial substance existing within a web of relationships, then depression, whatever its origin may be, inevitably will affect all parts of every person. If you agree with this, should there be any shame in seeking treatment from a variety of professionals?

7. If there should be no shame in needing medication in order to recover from (or just to live with) depression, why do you think so many believers feel guilty or inadequate because they need this help? Why do some even hide their illness from others?

8. Imagine that your best friend has just confided in you that he or she takes an antidepressant every day and has been doing so for some time. How would you respond? Would this knowledge affect your relationship either positively or negatively?

9. Based on what you've read in these first two chapters, what might be the most constructive and responsible way to proceed in terms of your own depression (or the depression of someone you care about)?

Brief Depression Scale

The following list of statements has been created to help you discern where you are in terms of depression. While it does not try to identify any causes or types of depression, it can be useful to you now, and it may prove useful to you after you have finished reading this book and/or participating in a discussion group.[17]

Directions: For each statement below, circle or underline the response that has described you over the past week.

1.	I often become bored.	Yes	No
2.	I often feel restless and fidgety.	Yes	No
3.	I feel in good spirits.	No	Yes
4.	I have more problems with memory than most.	Yes	No
5.	I can concentrate easily when reading the newspaper.	No	Yes
6.	I prefer to avoid social gatherings.	Yes	No
7.	I often feel downhearted or blue.	Yes	No
8.	I feel happy most of the time.	No	Yes
9.	I often feel helpless.	Yes	No
10.	I often feel worthless and ashamed of myself.	Yes	No
11.	I often wish I were dead.	Yes	No

Scoring:

Count 1 for each response in the first column. Scores of 4 or higher suggest that further evaluation should be pursued with a professional qualified to diagnose and/or treat depression.

© Harold G. Koenig, M.D., and Blackwell Publishing, Ltd.

CHAPTER 3

Do Real Christians Get Depressed?

There's a broken heart in every pew," wrote Joseph Parker, a British pastor in the nineteenth century. In the twenty-first century this reality hasn't changed, nor has there been any change in the sad fact that the church maintains a conspiracy of silence about depression, even though many believers through the ages have struggled with it. In this chapter you will meet some of them, both contemporary individuals and others who lived before the era of effective medical treatments for depression.

This chapter has two goals:

1. To encourage those who are depressed and those who love them that while depression may impair, even incapacitate for a while, it can be managed and it may inspire and empower a person to help others.
2. To open the eyes (and heart) of the church to the needs of the depressed in its midst and to erase the stigma so often attached (whether overtly or subtly) to this affliction.

Though treatment options have changed dramatically, for which we modern strugglers should be eternally grateful, there has been little change in the issues for believers affected by depression since the days of Job, who lived around 1500 B.C. As we journey with depression, we can be inspired by the "great cloud of witnesses" (Heb. 12:1) who remained faithful and kept going even when despair and darkness threatened to overwhelm them. Adorning this chapter you will find quotes from some of them, and we trust you'll be encouraged to know that even prophets, preachers, poets, kings, theologians, and media personalities have all walked the pathway you may be walking today. We also hope you will be encouraged to keep going and be inspired and enabled to break the silence that can exist between those who are depressed and those who love them, before it is too late.

The Caregiver

For twenty years Louanne had worked at an insurance agency. She took great pride in the high quality of her work. Although she had struggled with depression in the past, only recently had it interfered with her work. She was finding herself preoccupied at work with problems in her personal life, so much so that she was making mistakes. A few days before she came to see me (HK), she had been called into her employer's office for an error she had made on an important form that could not now be corrected. When he asked her what was wrong, Louanne had broken down in tears. "I felt so embarrassed," she told me, "but I just couldn't help it—I was just under too much pressure."

Louanne was having difficulty getting up in the morning to go to work, feeling like all of her energy was gone. She had not rested well at night for months. When she lay down to sleep at night, her mind raced from problem to problem. "I wake up real early, often around four o'clock," she reported. "As soon as I'm awake, those same problems seem to leap upon me and prevent me from falling asleep again."

She paused, then added, "I've lost my appetite too. Dropped ten pounds in the past three months. I don't mind losing the weight, but food doesn't even appeal to me anymore, and that's not like me."

"What kinds of things are making you feel stressed?" I asked.

"The question is where to start, Dr. Koenig. About five years ago my father was diagnosed with congestive heart failure. Three years ago his memory began to fade, which the doctor said was due to brain strokes he was having from his weak heart. My mother and I tried to manage him at home, but we couldn't handle his angry outbursts and heavy care needs. So about two years ago, we admitted him to a nursing home, and I became his health-care power of attorney. Suddenly it was up to me to make all his medical decisions.

"After he had been in that home for a few months, I concluded that he was not being taken care of very well. He was a difficult patient and would fight the nursing home staff when they tried to toilet or bathe him. Attempts were made by staff to restrain him physically, which sometimes caused bruises and skin tears on his arms. When I visited, I would often find him wet from his urine or soiled from stool that hadn't been cleaned up.

"So," Louanne paused and took a deep breath, "I decided to move him to another facility, but things haven't been much better there. It's been a constant battle with the nursing staff over his care. And none of my brothers or sisters—I have five of them—cares enough to help . . . just like always. I am the caregiver. Being the oldest daughter, I always took care of their kids, but this is different, very different."

"Tell me about your marriage," I said.

"Well," she replied, "that hasn't worked out the way I'd hoped either. Samuel is a wonderful, caring person, and I think we'd be okay if it weren't for Sam, Jr.—that's my stepson. He's seventeen now, and he takes everything I do for him for granted while refusing to accept me as a family member or as an authority in his life. His father sides with him every time there's a problem—which is most of the time these days. I feel absolutely helpless, at the mercy of this kid. He just sits in his room playing computer games with his heavy metal rock music playing as loud as he wants it. He's had two speeding tickets and an accident within the last year, so our auto insurance went sky high. He talks on the phone for hours with his girlfriend in Ohio.

"My husband doesn't confront him about any of these things, even though he was laid off from work a few months back, so the income from my job is all we have to go on. And now . . ." she started to cry quietly, "I can't even do my job right anymore. I used to be able to handle anything and everything, but now I just feel trapped and worthless . . . and worried. I'm even worried that I won't be able to afford your charges—I'm sorry—or medications if I need them. There simply isn't enough money to go around now, and I've been running up medical bills for the past few weeks with all kinds of aches and pains that I never had before. Sometimes," she paused again, "the pressure of it all just seems too much, and I just want out. I want it all to be over."

"You want your life to be over?"

"Yes."

"Have you ever tried to end your life?"

"No. Well, not really. Though last week, on my way home after another fight with my brother about his refusal to help with Dad, I had the strongest urge to just drive off the road into a tree."

"What kept you from doing that?"

"My faith, I guess," she said. "I know that suicide is never the right path for a Christian. So I drag myself out of bed, and I drag myself to

Why is light given to those in misery, and life to the bitter of soul, to those who long for death that does not come, who search for it more than for hidden treasure, who are filled with gladness and rejoice when they reach the grave? . . . For sighing comes to me instead of food; my groans pour out like water. . . . I have no peace, no quietness; I have no rest, but only turmoil.
—Job, blameless and upright man

I have had enough,
LORD. . . . Take my life;
I am no better than
my ancestors.
—Elijah,
Old Testament prophet

work. Then I drag myself home again, knowing full well that if Junior is home I'll have to put up with his chaos until it's late enough to drag myself to bed again . . . where I will lie awake rehearsing speeches I'd like to make but never will, or I worry about everything, sometimes for hours."

Although Louanne had seen several therapists intermittently over the years, she had not seen a psychiatrist before. One of the main reasons for her visit was to see if I, as a Christian psychiatrist, would recommend medications. She was seeing a certified counselor at her church, but this just wasn't enough. The church had always played a very large role in her life, and many of her friends and social support came from her church. She had turned her life over to Christ soon after graduating from high school, and this had been an enormous source of comfort for her. Although she didn't understand why God had allowed all of these negative stressors into her life, until recently she had clung to the hope that they were serving some purpose. Lately, however, she had realized that in the place where there was once only love for God, now there was mostly anger.

"Louanne," I said, toward the close of our session. "You have every reason to be depressed. Many people would have become depressed long ago, considering the pressures you face day-to-day. One reason you're having such a struggle now with the symptoms you mentioned is because over time your brain chemistry has become depleted from all this stress. You asked about medication. I believe, based on what you've said, that you would benefit from taking an antidepressant that will help restore the chemical balance you need in order not just to cope but to be yourself again. Also," I added, "I encourage you to keep seeing your counselor, especially since you have been gaining so much support from him."

Over the next three months, with medication and supportive counseling, Louanne gradually improved and her depression resolved.

The Bible Scholar

When J. B. Phillips was a child, his father pushed him to succeed because he knew his son was very talented. After Phillips entered the ministry, his anxieties about performing well for his earthly father manifested themselves in his feelings about his heavenly Father. Troubled by the concept of a demanding God and because his vocation as a man of God seemed to cause him so much stress, he quit his job as a curate in a church for a while.

However, over time the young clergyman was able to understand the root of his problematic relationship with God and deal with it. "Of all the false gods there is probably no greater nuisance than the 'god of one-hundred percent,'" he wrote. "After all, did not Christ say, 'Be ye perfect?' This one-hundred-percent standard . . . has taken the joy and spontaneity out of the Christian lives of many who dimly realize that what was meant to be a life of 'perfect freedom' has become an anxious slavery."[1]

Phillips's *Letters to Young Churches*, a translation of New Testament epistles, was published in 1947. Several years later, Phillips gave up his work with his church and for a time devoted his life to writing and speaking. His translation of the entire New Testament was immensely popular, especially in Great Britain and the United States, bringing instant fame and multiple speaking opportunities. It was a heady and dangerous time.

From 1955 to 1961 Phillips followed a hectic schedule, speaking often across the U.S. and in Great Britain. He was a highly successful radio broadcaster, writer, and public speaker. Finally, in 1961 the pressures of the author's touring schedule proved too much for him. After six years of frenetic travel and speaking, he was exhausted, depleted—in a word, depressed. "Without any particular warning the springs of creativity were suddenly dried up; the ability to communicate disappeared overnight and it looked as if my career as a writer and translator was over," he wrote.

> I know now, but had no idea then, that this was the first inkling of a condition known to the medical and psychiatric world as a depression, a condition that was to be with me for several years.
>
> After a few months, during which I was not entirely idle, I found the mental pain more than I felt I could bear and I went as a voluntary patient to a psychiatric clinic. . . .
>
> My reason for writing [about this] is that it may help someone else who is depressed and in mental pain. It may help simply to know that one whom the world would regard as successful and whose worldly needs are comfortably met can still enter this particular hell, and have to endure it for quite a long time.[2]

After his time in the clinic, Phillips experienced somewhat of a remission, and he was persuaded by evidently well-meaning folk to continue his translation work, this time taking on the Old Testament prophets Amos, Hosea, Micah, and Isaiah. His work, *Four Prophets*, was released in 1963. Yet again the success brought unexpected results when

The hardest thing of all to bear is what I can only describe as a nameless mental pain, which is, as far as I know, beyond the reach of any drug, and which I have tried in vain to describe to anyone. Other patients at the clinic knew it in varying degrees and bore it stoically. But it is so overwhelming that one can understand the temptation to suicide.
—J. B. Phillips, Bible translator

[I was struck] with such a dejection of spirits, as none but they who have felt the same, can have the least conception of. Day and night I was upon the rack, lying down in horror, and rising up in despair.
—William Cowper, hymn writer of "God Moves in Mysterious Ways"

he was overcome by a panic attack during a book signing, from which he was forced to depart.

Hospitalized again, the author attributed his breakdown to the pressure he had been under for years. He was unable to find any written Christian encouragement related to depression because it was

another of those forbidden subjects about which a tactful curtain of silence has for many years been drawn. . . . It would have been of inestimable comfort and encouragement to me in some of my darkest hours if I could have come across even one book written by someone who had experienced and survived the hellish torments of mind which can be produced . . . [an] almost unendurable sense of terror and alienation. . . .

The hardest thing of all to bear is what I can only describe as a nameless mental pain, which is, as far as I know, beyond the reach of any drug, and which I have tried in vain to describe to anyone. . . . But it is so overwhelming that one can understand the temptation to suicide.[3]

Ministry Cofounder

Jan Dravecky fell into the pit of depression as a result of exhaustion from unrelenting pressure from multiple stressors over a long period of time. With her husband, former major league baseball pitcher Dave Dravecky, Jan had launched a ministry to cancer victims. The publication of Dave's book *Comeback* had involved various media appearances and a book-signing tour. Dave's cancer, it seemed, was threatening the loss of his arm. Everything seemed to be happening so fast and with such intensity.

Jan's doctor tried to show her that her physical and psychological symptoms were consistent with the diagnosis of depression, but for a long time Jan would not accept the help her doctor offered. Instead, she tried to be strong. The following excerpt from her poignant book, *A Joy I'd Never Known*, describes the result of her attempt to will herself well:

I started crying again. I couldn't take much more. I just couldn't. I closed my drapes, pulled the covers up over my head, and sobbed. I stayed in bed, hour after hour, day after day, for the next three weeks, but I had lost any hopes that bed rest could cure me. . . .

I was starting to experience moments of utter darkness, dark days when I would feel a black fog come over everything in my life. Nothing looked good; life had lost all joy. As I lay there in one of these black emotional fogs with strange thoughts floating around in my mind, I

some of her (American) supporters: "Your missionary has begun to wonder why you have sent her no words of cheer, but yesterday there came a letter. . . . In your native land, surrounded by those who speak your mother tongue and whom you have known from infancy, you can scarcely have any idea how we in this foreign country look forward to the mail and how a chill, a feeling of despondency, will arise when there is nothing for us. The older missionaries say they are forgotten at home, that hardly anyone cares for them; and they tell us newcomers that it will be so with us in the lapse of time."[6]

Lottie Moon coped with her loneliness (and the unwillingness of her supporters to send her a female missionary for a colleague and a companion) by reading, walking along the shore or the beach, swimming, and maintaining flowers in a sort of makeshift garden.

During the winter of 1885–1886, the missionary felt a sense of depression for which she solicited prayer. "I feel my weakness and inability to accomplish anything without the aid of the Holy Spirit," she wrote. "Make special prayer for the outpouring of the Holy Spirit . . . that I may be clothed with power from on high by the indwelling of the Spirit in my heart."[7]

After returning to the United States in 1891, the exhausted and burned-out missionary allowed her sister to nurse her back to health. She was suffering a recurrent headache. "I have been so unmerciful to myself in China," she decided, "that I must call a halt now and take a needed rest." She followed this pattern for the rest of her life, often taking a month-long break from her work during the summer, during which she would relax and read.

After the Boxer Rebellion (1900–1901), the missionary fell into a severe depression because of the famine that she saw all around her in China. She refused to eat because she believed the girls whom she taught were starving. When friends tried to bring Lottie Moon back to the United States to recover her health, she died on the way, breathing her last breath in Japan.

The Politician

Long before he became a man, Abraham Lincoln was well acquainted with grief—and a candidate for depression. At the age of three he lost an infant brother. Six years later came a triple blow—the deaths of his aunt and uncle and his beloved mother, who had instilled in him a love for

You can scarcely have any idea how we in this foreign country look forward to the mail and how a chill, a feeling of despondency, will arise when there is nothing for us. The older missionaries say they are forgotten at home, that hardly anyone cares for them; and they tell us newcomers that it will be so with us in the lapse of time.
—Lottie Moon, missionary to China

God and books. Then twelve years later, when he was only eighteen, his only remaining sibling, a sister, died while giving birth. By the time Lincoln turned twenty-one, he had developed a variety of physical complaints in addition to a "look of gloom" arising from the fact that his left eye deviated upward. The doctors told him his illness was hypochondria—physical complaints with no medical basis—and they could not do anything about his eyes.

Lincoln's first recorded period of depression occurred during the spring of his twenty-fourth year when, after having performed well during wartime, he ran for public office and lost. His friends successfully campaigned for his appointment as the village postmaster. Although the job only lasted a few weeks, it soon led to his being hired as a surveyor's assistant. He was, finally, establishing a career path, which took on special importance since he was planning to marry his childhood love, Ann.

Two years later, however, the hammer fell again when Ann became ill and died of typhus. When Lincoln heard of his sweetheart's death, he became deeply depressed and wandered aimlessly among the hills and backcountry, refusing to eat or sleep. It did not help that he had been taught that death was often the direct act of God to punish the loved ones of the deceased person. Lincoln was eventually nursed back to health by Aunt Polly, who ministered to him physically and mentally until he had gone three weeks without a bout of "the chills."

Within a year Lincoln was seeing another woman, Mary, yet he still battled what had now become a chronic depression. Again campaigning for office, he wrote to Mary, "[I] have gotten my spirits so low that I feel I would rather be any place in the world than here. I really cannot endure the thought of staying here two weeks." Over time, the relationship waned.

A fourth period of depression occurred when Mary, the woman he would eventually wed, broke off their engagement on the day they were to be married, partly due to her fiancée's anxiety over the difference in their backgrounds—he being a poor, backwoods country type with only a single year of formal education while she was from a wealthy family. During this bout with depression, friends kept knives and razors away from Lincoln, and he did not carry a pocketknife for months, apparently fearful of his own suicidal tendencies.

At one point, Lincoln wrote: "I am now the most miserable man living. If what I feel were equally distributed to the whole human family, there would not be one cheerful face on earth. Whether I shall ever be better I cannot tell. I awfully forebode that I shall not. To remain as I am is impossible, I must die or be better, it appears to me."[8]

After Lincoln and Mary were married, they had problems and conflicts because he was an introvert and she was an extrovert. However, there were no further depressive episodes for twenty years, partly because Lincoln had successfully run for office and was preoccupied with governmental matters. This was particularly true during the final years of his life when he was president during a period of grave crisis in the United States.

In the midst of this national crisis, the couple's young son, William, died, and depression returned with a vengeance. Though affairs of state demanded Lincoln's attention, the bereaved father became socially distant and often shut himself in a room for hours. Amazingly, during this time the heartbroken man reconciled himself with God, returning to the faith of his childhood, now with a much different, deeper understanding. Two years later, on April 14, 1865, an assassin's bullet ended the long and painful journey of Abraham Lincoln, whom many consider this country's greatest president.[9]

Contemporary Christian Media Personality

Sheila Walsh was born and grew up in Ayr, Scotland, where her family attended a local Baptist church. It was at that church that the girl first became intrigued by music, especially devotional Christian music and Celtic sounds. As a teenager she loved the pop-rock music she and her friends heard on the radio, and she began to express her faith through songs. Walsh was the only Christian in her high school class, and she wanted to communicate the truth to her peers in a way they would understand. This was the desire that launched her musical career.

With her God-given talents and friends like pop star Cliff Richard, Walsh worked with Youth for Christ, the Billy Graham Crusades, and other youth ministries as they offered hope to thousands in the British Isles. She took the Gospel to a new place when the BBC asked her to host "The Rock Gospel Show," marking Britain's first prime-time Christian program. It wasn't long until her gifts took her across the waters to the United States, where she was signed to a major label and acknowledged in the 1980s as International Artist of the Year by the Gospel Music Association. Subsequent Grammy and Dove nominations helped the recording artist earn a place among Christian music's most respected artists. Walsh's success as a contemporary Christian music artist led to her cohosting Pat Robertson's Christian Broadcast Network show *The 700*

How long, O LORD? Will you forget me forever? How long will you hide your face from me? How long must I wrestle with my thoughts and every day have sorrow in my heart?
—David, King of Israel

Club. She also hosted a daily talk show on the Family Channel called *Heart to Heart.* The hosting duties for both of those shows lasted from 1987 to 1992. However, despite the success (or perhaps partly due to it) Walsh attained during this time, she fell into depression. Overworked with many commitments, she suffered burnout, frustration, bitterness, and anger. Eventually, she took a leave of absence from her television duties, checked into a psychiatric hospital, and was ultimately diagnosed with clinical depression.

During her hospitalization Walsh relished what she called a "companionship of brokenness" with her fellow patients and achieved a new, more enlightened viewpoint of depression and of her life as a Christian. She drew upon her struggle with depression to write her autobiographical and inspirational book, *Honestly,* which was published in 1996 and became a bestseller. This book describes, as forthrightly as any Christian book on the subject of depression, the variety of issues that often plague people with depression including anxiety, fear of intimacy, perfectionism, sadness, anger, and shame. The author speaks transparently about her disappointment with herself, from her divorce to her withdrawal from the media limelight. She heard many comments, learned of unfounded rumors being spread about her, and received many letters condemning her at a time when she most needed support from her former friends.

"Failure can be an awesome teacher if we invite Christ into the process," she wrote. "It was good for me that my friends distanced themselves, because it ultimately forced me to face my terrible fear of rejection and bring it to Jesus. . . . But at the time, the silence I encountered added to my feelings of utter hopelessness. I had failed, therefore I was a failure. The hopelessness I felt was so pervasive that I ignored the calls of one old friend who wanted to come see me. I felt so ashamed that I could not look at anyone." [10]

Do Real Christians Get Depressed?

The answer to this question should be clear enough by now. Not all Christians become depressed, but some do. In fact, quite a few do. Our belief is that far more believers struggle with depression than the relative silence of the church on this issue might indicate.

As we said earlier and the cases of this chapter clearly demonstrate, depression is no respecter of persons. Depression is also no respecter of age. It afflicts older adults, especially when they become ill or physically disabled, although research has shown that its incidence among the elderly is actually less than that in those who are younger.[11] Among persons aged sixty-five or over who are healthy enough to live at home, the rate of serious depression is less than 1 percent compared to about 4 percent in persons aged eighteen to forty-four.

Depression is also common among those under age eighteen. Depression is present in 0.4 to 2.5 percent of children, 0.4 to 8.3 percent of adolescents, and nearly 10 percent of high school students. Depression is increasing at "an alarming rate," according to the National Mental Health Association. Unfortunately, 70 to 80 percent of depressed teens do not receive treatment.[12]

This last fact helps explain why suicide has become the third leading cause of death for young people age fifteen to twenty-four (and the sixth leading cause of death for children five to fifteen years old). Each year in the United States almost five thousand young people ages fifteen to twenty-four kill themselves. The rate of suicide for this age group has nearly tripled since 1960. Suicide is the second leading cause of death among college-age youth, even though as many as 80 percent usually give some indication to others that they are considering suicide.[13]

This was true in the case of Bill, the son of Dr. and Mrs. George Nichols. After Bill's death, Dr. Nichols, now retired, devoted a significant portion of the rest of his medical career to educating anyone who would listen to the signs and symptoms of this sometimes deadly disorder.

"We lost our son, Bill, to an unrecognized depressive illness, which led to his suicide," Dr. Nichols wrote.

> That was in 1985. We still miss him. He was a fine young man. He fought bravely, but silently and alone. Bill was working two thousand miles away when he became depressed. He showed the classic signs of depression, but I had no chance to see them. Some people suspected that things were not right with Bill, but no one seemed to know what those signs meant, or what to do, and Bill's life ended.
>
> Many people still think of depression not as a treatable sickness, but as a personal weakness, a lack of willpower, a failure of one's religious faith, or a shameful failure of family upbringing. Many of my patients have a deep religious faith, to which they have naturally turned for help with their emotional distress, not realizing that these distressed feelings may be due to a biochemical imbalance rather than to a lack of faith. While it is true that depression may involve social stresses, failure, loss, and isolation, we also know that sometimes it just pops up

He has besieged me and surrounded me with bitterness and hardship. He has made me dwell in darkness like those long dead. He has walled me in so I cannot escape; he has weighed me down with chains. Even when I call out or cry for help, he shuts out my prayer. He has barred my way with blocks of stone; he has made my paths crooked.
—Jeremiah,
Old Testament prophet

Causeless depression cannot be reasoned with, nor can David's harp charm it away by sweet discoursings. [We may] as well fight with the mist as with this shapeless, undefinable, yet all-beclouding hopelessness. . . . The iron bolt which so mysteriously fastens the door of hope and holds our spirits in gloomy prison, needs a heavenly hand to push it back.
—Charles Spurgeon, English preacher

when people are not having any problems at all. By most standards, they ought to be on top of the world. But they are in the slime pit of despair, without any apparent reason.

This is what I didn't really understand well enough until I began to study it more deeply after Bill's death. Like pneumonia and high blood pressure, depression happens in good families, and it happens in bad families. It happens to religious people, and to nonreligious people. It happens to all kinds of people, even children, all over the world. It is not shameful to be sick, but old misperceptions too often prevent people with depressive sickness from being recognized and treated and rescued, even by those who ought to know better. And that *is* truly shameful.

Not everyone who is depressed looks sad; sometimes they laugh and may even deny that they feel "depressed." In any case, it can be a tragic mistake to delay treatment by talking, listening, reasoning, advising, or trying to restore hope—things that are good in other situations. That counseling can come after recovery from the sickness.

Initially, a different kind of help is needed to restore those chemical connections in the brain. You may be the only person who will ever suspect that John or Mary is sick with depression, so don't decide to watch and wait! Act! Act on your suspicions by seeing that John or Mary gets to a physician right away. Take him or her to the doctor yourself if that's the only way you can be sure they will go, and let the doctor decide what's wrong and how to intervene.

Occasionally treatment fails, nothing works, and this makes everyone sad. But most of the time (60 to 80 percent) people treated with a combination of antidepressant medicine and talk (psychotherapy) begin to show improvement within the first few weeks. Eventually, they return to their usual selves.

If the depression is not treated medically, recovery may occur. But if it does, usually it is only after months of misery—not only for the person who is depressed, but for everyone around him or her—family, friends, and colleagues at work. (People with depression, with all their complaints and gloom, are often a "pain in the neck" to those around them, especially when others don't recognize the depression.) And there is always the risk of suicide in 10 to 15 percent of people with this disorder, because the sick brain is too impaired to make good decisions, or to see reality except through a muddled haze.

Suicide is usually a shocking surprise to the family and to friends who only then realize how serious things were. Over and over the stunned survivors ask, "What went wrong?"—not understanding that the person was sick. It wasn't just stress, or a wrong choice. It was an illness called depression, outside one's self-control, capable of over-

whelming any of us. People in great despair sometimes try to free themselves from depression through intense and sincere spiritual effort. Well-
meaning friends may compound their depressed friends' agony by telling
them that some discipline or experience they have not yet had will lift
them from the pit. Such methods are wrong-headed because they fail to
treat the cause of the illness. They are also dangerous because, in failing,
they prolong the sickness and risk a fatal termination.

Do real Christians get depressed? You bet they do. My own perspective is that my patients, including my Christian patients, do best
when they adopt exactly the same attitude toward the chemical solutions that modern medicine has provided for their depression as they
have for the medicines they take for hypertension, diabetes, or pneumonia. Seeing people rediscover purpose, meaning, and joy through
this means makes it clear to me that these medical interventions should
be viewed as God's allies, for if I understand his Word correctly, he
desires these very same things [a sense of purpose, meaning, and joy]
for all who trust in him.[14]

Questions for Reflection

1. What is the net result of having read through the cases in this
   chapter?
   ☐ I feel encouraged.
   ☐ I feel discouraged.
   ☐ I feel afraid.
   ☐ I feel hopeful.

2. What common themes did you notice in these stories?

3. Try to express in a sentence how these examples affect your
   understanding of faith as it relates to depression.

4. How did these examples affect your understanding of depression
   (your own or the depression of someone you care about)?

5. If you agree that there has been a "conspiracy of silence" in the
   church about depression among people of faith, why do you think
   this has been true?

6. If a friend confided in you that he or she was considering suicide,
   what would you say or do? Suggestion: If studying in a group,
   have several pairs of people role-play this situation and then
   discuss it together.

7. Do you think it is easier or more difficult for Christians to seek medical help when depressed?

8. If your Christian friend were seeking treatment for depression, what would you do or say to encourage him or her?

9. Project yourself to a year from now: Envision God using your experience with depression to bless or help others. Describe in a general sense what that would look like. What would you be doing? Where? With or for whom? What would be your goals?

10. Write your responses in your journal along with a simple prayer asking God's help in realizing this vision of your future. Share any part of your responses to these last two questions with your group, if you wish to do so.

Lifesaving Questions

By learning to ask the right questions and then following up any clues the depressed person provides in response, you may be able to engage that person in a lifesaving conversation about the effect that his or her depression is having—emotionally, physically, cognitively, and even spiritually. Here are some sample questions about various areas and suggestions about how to follow up.

Depressed Mood

"You sound kind of down. How are you?"

"You seem discouraged. Are things okay?"

"Lately have you been especially worried about something?

"Do you find yourself more easily upset these days than usual?"

Listen for gloomy or pessimistic remarks, such as:

"What difference does it make?"

"I just don't care anymore."

Respond further, for example:

"Well, it makes a difference to me as your friend. But I wonder, have you been feeling this way long?"

"Sometimes people who feel this way don't even care if they hurt themselves; for example, they may drive recklessly or abuse alcohol or drugs. Do you think you could do such things?"

Remember that depression can be masked by physical ailments. With this in mind, you might ask, "Have you been feeling well?"

Expect to hear a litany of recently developed symptoms, such as headache, backache, stomachache, constipation, chronic pain. Take care not to invalidate this pain, since it is real to the depressed person, but you might ask, "Do you think this might be a bad disease? What does your doctor say?"

One overarching thing to keep in mind is that depressed people, given a listening ear, will complain at length about a personal problem, loss, or sense of failure. If you wish to help, be prepared to hear this litany of distress over and over again. They are, most likely, either unaware of this repetition, or testing the level of your love, or both, so it will not help to try to shut this off, as many do, with comments like: "You shouldn't feel that way."

A better response might be, "I'm sorry you're having these troubles. If I were having them, I might feel pretty confused (angry/upset/down/worried, etc.). How do these things make you feel inside?" Or, "I'm sorry you're having these troubles, and if I had the power I would make them go away. Can we think of a way that I can help you with them?"

Loss of Pleasure and Interests

If the person's interest was a creative hobby: "Have you been doing any woodworking (knitting, photography, etc.) lately?"

If the answer indicates the person has lost interest in the hobby you might say: "You know, you have a real talent for (_____). I really enjoy your work." (If applicable: "Your creations occupy places of honor in my home. When do you think you'll have the energy to take _____ up again?")

If the person followed sports: "Still keeping up with the Broncos?" (or any other sports team).

If he or she enjoyed recreation: "How's your golf game?" (or whatever activity). If cooking or gardening, perhaps you might bring along a new cookbook or gardening book or catalog to see if you can engage the person in conversation about such things.

If it seems that the person has become withdrawn or feels isolated, you might ask: "Have you been to church lately?" or "Seen your old friend, Jim, lately?" or "Been out to see any movies lately?" Or, if you think this may help, you might offer: "_____ and I are going out to dinner and a movie Saturday. We'd love for you to come along as our guest."

Feelings of Worthlessness and Excessive Guilt

These feelings are often expressed in self-deprecating remarks or endless apologies for even the most insignificant of perceived wrongs. An appeal to the mind—as in: "That's really not so bad; everybody does that"—likely will not help much as this is primarily a matter of the heart.

Instead, you might say something like: "It's clear that you feel guilty about and responsible for (whatever it is). And it's also clear that nothing anyone says can change the way you feel, because we've all tried, and the feelings are still there. So instead of trying to talk you out of feeling guilty, I'd like to say something else. I love you (care very much about you). Maybe you did do (whatever—or did not do whatever) and something really bad happened for which you feel responsible. So, just for the moment, let's agree that you *are* guilty. You're guilty of being a human being, of not knowing everything, etc. Even so, I still love you. What's more, I forgive you, my friend. As far as I'm concerned, you are forgiven."

Keep in mind that feelings of worthlessness can also lie behind such symptoms as personal sloppiness (in a person who was previously well-dressed or well-groomed). Poor self-care or housekeeping may be evident. Be aware that your effort to help—as in swooping in with a crew of helpers to clean up the house without prior permission—may hurt rather than help a depressed person. Ahead of time, you might say: "I understand that sometimes when a person's really discouraged, things like the laundry (or dishes or general housework) can just get left undone. I'm sure that you'll get better, but I'm wondering if you'd mind if I helped with (whatever it is)."

Sluggishness or Agitation

"You seem to be moving (or speaking) more slowly than usual. Is that the way you feel, as if everything's in slow motion?"
Or, if it applies, "You seem nervous or restless today. Is that the way you've been feeling?"

Fatigue, Loss of Energy

"Have you been feeling really tired lately?"
"Having trouble getting going in the morning?"

If the answer is "yes," then you might inquire if he or she has been working hard on something. (Note: The depressed mind works nonstop on one's problems—whether real or perceived makes little difference—which is one reason why most depressed people are perpetually exhausted.)

Trouble Thinking, Concentrating, Deciding

"Sometimes when I feel stressed, I have trouble keeping my mind on what I'm doing, from reading the paper to watching television to driving. Can you identify with that?"
"Sometimes when I feel pressured, I have a really hard time making decisions. Do you know what I mean?"

"When I'm really worried, I can hardly think straight. Ever felt that way?"

Change in Weight

If you can see that the person has lost or gained a significant amount of weight within a relatively short amount of time, it may be tricky to bring it up, but you might say something like, "You know, every day I get spammed by e-mails advertising weight-loss programs. I don't usually pay attention to them, but I was thinking of investigating the XYZ program. Have you heard of that?"

Change in Sleep Patterns

"Lately, I've been having trouble getting to sleep at night. Maybe it's too much caffeine, or maybe too much on my mind. Have you ever had a problem like that?"

"I've been waking up really early lately, and then I just lie there waiting for the alarm to go off. Do you know of any methods for overcoming this sort of thing?"

Recurrent Thoughts of Death or Suicide

This, too, can be a very difficult subject, but as this chapter has shown, it's one of a few subjects that you may not be able to return to later should you put if off now. (Note: We'll have more to say about suicide prevention in chapter 11, "Love: The Crucial Role of Family and Friends.") One way to broach the subject indirectly is to note something on the news that relates to suicide, as when a famous person takes his own life or a terminally ill person chooses physician-assisted suicide. You might ask, "Did you hear about XYZ (singer, actor, etc.) who jumped off a bridge (or whatever) the other day? I wonder how a person with so much to live for could choose to end it like that?" Or "Did

you hear about that man/woman in Michigan who asked the doctor to help her die because she couldn't face living with Alzheimer's?"

Or you could say something like, "The other day I was reading the story of Job in the Old Testament. Did you know that he got so low that he cursed the day of his birth, as if he wished he'd never been born? And God didn't even strike him with lightning for talking that way!" If the person interacts with this, follow his or her lead, but be sure to find out if he or she has also been feeling this same way.

If the person is already speaking about death, dying, or suicide, you might take a more direct route, as in, "You sound discouraged enough to hurt yourself. Would you please tell me what you mean?"

If the person admits to self-destructive or suicidal ideas, you cannot just walk away. For one thing, the person is taking a risk of letting you inside his or her heart. So beyond the ideas we provide in chapter 11, you need to communicate at least the following: "I want you to know that I consider it a privilege that you've given me this glimpse into your heart. Thank you for trusting me that much. And because I want to honor that trust, I need to know how serious you are, because I, for one, would really miss you if something like this happened. I mean, it's one thing to think about or be tempted to do something. It's another to actually do it. For example, do you have a plan of how you would do this?" If the answer is "yes," the plans are specific, and the person is determined, then you have no choice but to stay with the person until you are sure that he or she cannot follow through, even to the point of involuntary hospitalization if necessary. Though your hospitalized friend may hate you for a while, we guarantee he or she will thank you later.[15]

~∂~——————————————————————————

CHAPTER 4

Ten Myths and Misconceptions

We believe there are many myths and misconceptions related to depression, including its causes and treatments. These often contribute, both in society and the church, to misunderstandings about people with depression, how to help them, or even how to simply relate to them. We offer the following representative list, knowing full well that no list can hope to describe all the myths and misconceptions related to such a complex disorder.

Myth 1: You're depressed because you want to be depressed.

We can only imagine what Charles Spurgeon might have said to the suggestion that he was depressed because he wanted to be. Undoubtedly the best-known English preacher of his day, Spurgeon's collected sermons fill sixty-three volumes—the largest set of books by a single author in the history of Christianity. This great man of God, who struggled with depression for years, once wrote, "There are dungeons beneath the castle of despair."[1] In other words, Spurgeon's view was that he had suffered with depths of depression even deeper than those described by John Bunyan in *Pilgrim's Progress*.

It is possible for people to become accustomed to being depressed or to become so familiar with it that change is threatening. In other words, it is possible to become "addicted to sadness." I (DB) coined this phrase as a result of reading Gerald G. May's book, *Addiction and Grace,* in which the author describes the various components of addictions and how the grace of God can heal them. I realized that the five characteristics of addiction[2] described by this author could relate not only to substances and behaviors but also to sadness—my sadness. *All* of them have been true of me at one time or another during my journey with depression:

1. *Tolerance.* Once you are adjusted to your attachment to whatever it is, you need more of it to achieve the same effect. As my sadness became a chronic state, I seemed to need more of it to maintain my equilibrium of unhappiness. It was relatively easy to identify things to be unhappy about or to create them when necessary.

2. *Withdrawal symptoms.* Because I had become habituated to sadness as a state of existence, the prospect of exchanging that state for another, even happiness, caused anxiety. In situations that had previously produced pleasure, I often managed to turn them into stressful events by concocting reasons to not enjoy whatever it was we were planning to do. For example, if we were going fishing, I would have to know every last detail of the fishing regulations, or I would focus on the possibility that someone might drown or get into the poison ivy. Later, I would chastise myself for ruining another family outing.

3. *Self-deception.* Although my increasing depression was apparent to others, I denied that I needed help. I even managed to turn it around, for example, by thinking or saying that the only help I needed was for people to either accept me as I was or leave me alone. Naturally, I gravitated away from my critics and toward those who allowed me to continue down the path I was on. In other words, I managed to convince some to support my addiction in a variety of ways. The psychological term for this dynamic is *co-dependence.*

4. *Loss of willpower.* "One part of the will sincerely wants to be free," Dr. May wrote. "Another part wants to continue the addictive behavior. At certain points, it even encourages making resolutions to stop. It knows such resolutions are likely to fail, and when they do, the addictive behavior will have a stronger foothold than ever."[3] I (DB) distinctly recall standing in front of the church I was pastoring late on New Year's Eve 1978, resolving that the coming year would be different. It was. It was worse.

5. *Distortion of attention.* I became so preoccupied with my own sadness that my energies were consumed by it, to the detriment of relationships with my family and others, including God, since

one cannot love anyone without paying attention to that person. To the same degree that my attention was focused on myself, I was unable to love others.

Some might say the pattern just described proves that depression is a matter of deliberate choice. Based on what we've experienced and observed, we would say that while some conscious choices are certainly made along the way, most of the dynamics are unconscious rather than deliberate. Not all depressed people will become addicted to sadness, but none of those who do so have willfully chosen to subject themselves to something that will ultimately control their lives any more than a drug addict intended to become addicted when he smoked his first joint.

We agree that some people seem to hold on to their depression because it elicits sympathy, attention, or care from those around them. These cases, however, are not very common, and many of them may also represent unconscious choices. Most people who are depressed aren't depressed because they want to be. Most Christians who are depressed long to joyfully fulfill the purpose for which God has called them out of darkness into his marvelous light.

In fact, depression is often more difficult for Christians because the pain they feel is compounded by guilt that they cannot be who they long to be in Christ. Their guilt is further compounded by their knowledge that they ought not to feel guilty, since in Christ they are forgiven. The whole experience is like a spiral staircase leading nowhere, while the effort to progress leaves them exhausted—physically, emotionally, and spiritually. Having reached this state, pressed down by life, their hearts hammered by well-meaning friends, people who are depressed could no more choose to be happy than they could choose not to feel pain if they banged their finger with a real hammer.

Most Christians who are depressed long to joyfully fulfill the purpose for which God has called them out of darkness into his marvelous light.

Myth 2: You can beat depression with willpower.

This myth could be considered the flip side of the first one, but it was my strategy (HK). I was determined to find my own way out of the emotional mess I was in. I would listen to no one and rejected the advice of friends and family. I figured that I could do it entirely on my own through sheer self-mastery. I would pull myself up by my own bootstraps. It didn't work; it never does, because it can't. John Donne said, "No man is an island, entire of it self."[4] We were created to live in relationship, which includes receiving input and guidance from others, since no one person has complete knowledge from all perspectives on a situation.

Over time I became increasingly isolated, withdrawn into a fantasy world of my own creation. This led to my being expelled from medical school, living on the streets, and nearly going insane. It took years of senseless wandering and a string of broken relationships before I was finally rescued by coming to know the Lord. He gave me the power to overcome my problems, a direction for my life, and a caring faith community that I allowed to support and guide me. Willpower wasn't enough. The force of my emotional demons was just too strong for me. I needed God and his people to get me straight.

When we choose to align ourselves with God's will, he gives us both the will and the ability to work for his good pleasure (see Phil. 2:12–13), which is that ultimately all things in heaven and earth will be brought under the lordship of Jesus Christ (see Eph. 1:3–10). How our lives witness to his power, including his power over depression, is part of that process. We cannot will ourselves well; we can only willfully entrust ourselves and our needs to the one who understands us best, asking him to enable and empower us to live with our depression in a way that will honor him.

Myth 3: You're depressed because of unconfessed sins.

In his preface to *Why Do Christians Shoot Their Wounded?* Christian psychiatrist Dr. Dwight Carlson wrote, "In my experience, Christians are intolerant, if not prejudiced, against individuals with emotional difficulties. Most view all such problems as due to personal sin. Some well-known Christian authors have fueled the fires of stigma and judgment toward those suffering with emotional illness."[5]

To continue the military analogy, we think the church should function more like a MASH unit. We should be patching up the wounded so they can get back to the front lines to engage the enemy, perhaps even more effectively than before due to the insights and wisdom they've gained into the enemy's strategies and methods.

Instead, in the church we too often use words to rub salt in people's wounds. Based on our experience and observation, well-meaning Christians have the distressing habit of saying hurtful things to people in pain, including people with depression. For example, if you're depressed, you've been told at least once (perhaps many times) that the root of your depression is unconfessed sin. Some counseling methods are based on helping people identify (or dredge up from their unconscious) sins they must confess.

While spiritual disciplines, including confession and prayer, may be helpful in alleviating some symptoms of depression,[6] the myth we're dealing with here is based on a superficial understanding of sin and its consequences. The biblical view is that sin is a part of our nature (even after we become believers) and that our sins are proof of this fact. This is why the apostle Paul could so accurately describe in Romans 7:14–8:1 the basic inner conflict between our new nature (which comes from God, gives life to our souls, and enables us to become more Christlike) and our old nature (which still wants its own selfish way). One might even think, based on his words, that the situation *depresses* Paul: "Wretched man that I am! Who will set me free from the body of this death?"

Thankfully, the answer to that question is the same for all who believe, including those with depression: "Thanks be to God through Jesus Christ our Lord. . . . There is therefore now no condemnation for those who are in Christ Jesus." The only antidote to our sins or the guilt relating to them is total and absolute reliance on the fact that our faith in Christ places us "in him," as a result of which we are justified before God.

In other words, the only solution to the problem of our sins is not to try to root them out one by one. This is an impossible task since we are unaware of many of our sins, from pride to prejudice to envy to whatever. The only solution to our *sins* is provided in the solution to our *sin*— that the Lord God has laid upon Jesus Christ the iniquity of all who trust in him (see Isa. 53:6; Eph. 2:8–9).

In relation to the myth in question, the main problem for depressed believers is not so much their unconfessed sins as their guilt feelings over sins that God has already forgiven combined with an inability to personally grasp the meaning of Christ's death in relation to their sin. Depressed Christians are sometimes so *painfully aware of their sins* that this is all they can focus on. A single-minded focus like this is called an obsession. When a person is in this state, he or she may be unable to reflect rationally about this matter until the biochemistry causing such self-deprecation has been repaired. Thus, it surely will not help to state that he or she is being disobedient for not simply accepting God's forgiveness, which could make the person feel he or she is more of a sinner than anyone else. Such allegations can only further hurt a wounded

Depressed Christians are sometimes so painfully *aware of their sins* that it *becomes an obsession.*

heart, leaving the person feeling more disconnected from the Christian community.

Myth 4: If you're depressed, you're just feeling sorry for yourself.

People without depression often glibly tell those who are depressed to stop feeling sorry for themselves and snap out of it. These advisors don't want to be burdened with the struggles of others. They don't want to be reminded that life isn't one long "climb, climb, up sunshine mountain; faces all aglow," with God handing out smiley face stickers along the way. Many Christians want to believe that because they are "good people" they deserve a worry-free, pain-free life, but of course their assumption is wrong.

Job's friends also had this mistaken assumption. Their entire system of religion was threatened by the fact that Job, an upright man, had experienced such horrendous losses. Their thinking went like this: If such bad things could happen to Job, as virtuous as he is, then worse things surely could happen to us. Job had this fear in view when he said to them, "A despairing man should have the devotion of his friends, even though he forsakes the fear of the Almighty [which Job had not done]. But my brothers are as undependable as intermittent streams. . . . Now you too have proved to be of no help; you see something dreadful and are afraid" (Job 6:14–15, 21).

Potential helpers will be burdened with the struggles of those who are depressed if they choose to support and encourage those who hurt, because this kind of involvement (in order to be done well) makes demands on a helper's time and energy. It also immerses the helper in a process that ultimately may challenge his or her presuppositions and bring change *to the helper's mind and heart*. For some people, the possibility that change leading to growth in *themselves* might be brought about by interacting with the depressed person is quite threatening.

Usually people who promulgate myths like this one only have experience dealing with minor problems, not with a history of repeated major losses, abuses, or tragedies that have drained life of purpose and meaning. In addition, they probably don't have a biological predisposition to depression, which can magnify the weight of such problems a thousand times. Of such critics, Charles Spurgeon said, "Any fool can sing in the day. When the cup is full, man draws inspiration from it; when wealth rolls in abundance around him, any man can sing to the praise of a God who gives a plenteous harvest. . . . But the skillful singer is he who can sing when there is not a ray of light to read by . . . who sings from his heart, and not from a book that he can see, because he has no means of reading, save from that inward book of his own living spirit, whence notes of gratitude pour out in songs of praise. . . . It is not natural to sing in trouble. . . . Songs in the night come only from God; they are not in the power of man."[7]

Sometimes people who believe this myth say, "A lot of people have it worse than you," which is a way of keeping those who hurt at arm's length, refusing to validate their pain. Or some people may add, "In fact, I have it worse than you. Let me tell you all the bad things that have happened to me . . . and *I'm* not depressed!" This response makes it clear that either they are projecting their own self-pity onto the depressed person or they really don't care about the depressed person's needs. Either way, as Job said to his friends, this type of "comfort" is of no help whatsoever.

A parallel statement is less direct but equally unhelpful. It goes something like this: "Although I haven't experienced a situation like yours in reality, I have faced it theoretically." For example, a fellow pastor once told me (DB) that he had already faced the possibility of his own son's death (though his son was in perfect health at that moment). This was his way of saying that if I were as spiritually mature as he, I would cut the self-pity party and get on with living. I don't recall responding, for what can one say to such a claim? Today I suppose I might note that virtual reality isn't the same as reality, and there is no way he could know what it is like by simply imagining it. When we are depressed it can be difficult to know how to properly respond to the hurtful things people say to us, but it's best not to let comments like these get us down. Remember that almost without exception, people who say such things don't have any idea what they're talking about.

Myth 5: Depressed believers have weak faith.

People who haven't experienced depression can't imagine how this disorder makes it difficult to concentrate, sucks away energy and motivation, draws people into themselves, and paralyzes action. For these reasons, it should not be surprising that depressed Christians have difficulty praying, having devotions, or going to church.

For some, the experience of depression engenders deeper spiritual insight because their pain forces them to reach out to God in a new way.

In his excellent book, *The Masks of Melancholy*, Christian psychiatrist John White says that, based on his experience, mere devotional reading should actually be discouraged for depressed people because it might degenerate into something spiritually unhealthy and unhelpful. He is referring to the tendency of depressed believers to perceive all manner of exhortations often found in devotional books as messages from God or in some way having special application to their own situation. When such admonishments have to do with what is perceived by many as "the normal Christian life"[8] of being filled with the Spirit, exhibiting the fruit of the Spirit, rising above one's problems, and so forth, the depressed Christian feels indicted, not inspired toward greater Christlikeness.

By contrast, White says that solid, inductive Bible study should be encouraged (if the person is actually able to concentrate), with oversight by a pastor or pastoral counselor. "Years ago, when I was seriously depressed," he explains, "the thing that saved my own sanity was a dry-as-dust grappling with Hosea's prophecy. I spent weeks, morning by morning, making meticulous notes, checking historical allusions in the text. Slowly I began to sense the ground under my feet growing steadily firmer. I knew without any doubt that healing was constantly springing from my struggle to grasp the meaning of the prophecy."[9]

Critical observers sometimes conclude that a depressed person's inability to engage in spiritual activities is the *cause* of his or her depression, when it is actually a *result* of depression. When well-meaning helpers become critics of a depressed believer's spiritual life, as did Job's advisors, they add to the burden rather than lighten it. This is not only unhelpful, but it may be displeasing to God, who held Job's friends accountable for the way they treated him.

For many believers through the ages who have struggled with depression, their experience has engendered deeper spiritual insight because their pain has forced them to reach out to God in a new way. Rather than being evidence of weak faith, depression has been, historically, a common route to spiritual growth and insight for many of our spiritual guides, including one named Martin Luther.

Born to German parents who were stern disciplinarians, Luther grew up with strong impressions about sin and punishment. On occasion his father beat him, and once his mother whipped him until he bled for stealing a nut. Evidently the boy was also stubborn and willful enough outside the home that once he was whipped by a teacher fifteen times for misbehaving.

After joining the scholarly Augustinian order of monks, being ordained as a priest, and making a pilgrimage (on foot) to Rome, the budding theologian became increasingly anxious about what he perceived to be God's chastising of him for sin. He would spend hours in confessional booths.

Upon entering the monastery, Luther attempted to subdue his sinful pride by taking on menial tasks such as sweeping the floor, but his conscience still haunted him. In order to cleanse himself from sin and earn God's grace, he punished himself by practicing ascetic activities such as fasting and keeping to himself in his room for long periods of time. Of this practice he wrote: "I tormented myself to death to procure peace with God for my troubled heart and my agitated conscience; but I was surrounded by horrible darkness, and could find peace nowhere."[10] At one point Luther became extremely depressed and overwhelmed by guilt, so he locked himself in his monk's cell for several days. When another monk knocked on the door and heard no sound inside, he broke the door open and saw the penitent stretched out on the floor, seemingly unconscious.

Not long thereafter, as a result of studying the Scriptures, Luther challenged his church over the selling of indulgences—forgiveness of sin in exchange for money—because it had become clear to him that no man had the power to forgive sin. The lines drawn, a battle for truth began during which the reformer experienced times of great inner conflict when he could envision the devil in the room with him, urging him to recant and return to the fold of Rome. Once their dialogue seemed so real that the unrepentant protester finally threw an inkwell at the personage he believed to be before him. The inkwell hit the wall of his study, splattering ink all over it, running down to the floor, and spreading in an ever-widening pool, mirroring the ever-widening impact that his teachings enjoyed despite great persecution and pressure at home and abroad.

Having left the priesthood, at age forty Luther married a former nun who was sixteen years younger than he. Their marriage produced six children. The near death of his first son during the plague forced Luther to contemplate the mysteries of life and death in a new way. Yet perhaps the greatest emotional crisis of the reformer's adult life came when the couple's second child, Elizabeth, died, leaving the mother struggling with guilt and the father crushed and despondent for some time.

One of the fruits of all of Luther's struggles was a hymn that he gave to his friends a year after Elizabeth's death. Its words still ring true today, nearly five hundred years after they were penned:

A mighty Fortress is our God, a bulwark never failing;
Our Helper He, amid the flood of mortal ills prevailing.
For still our ancient foe, doth seek to work us woe;
His craft and pow'r are great; and, armed with cruel hate,
On earth is not his equal.

Let goods and kindred go, this mortal life also;
The body they may kill; God's truth abideth still,
His Kingdom is forever.[11]

Anyone who knows the life and times of Martin Luther would agree that in spite of the fact that he struggled with depression throughout much of his adult life, the word *weak* does not apply either to him or to his faith.

Myth 6: It's easy to tell when you are depressed.

Depression is not easy to identify, especially for the person who is depressed. One of the hallmark symptoms of severe depression is that people lose the ability to recognize that they have an illness that needs treatment. They believe they are dealing with reality for which there is no possible change or cure. This sense of helplessness and hopelessness is a lie that the vulnerable depressed person easily accepts.

Many people also have difficulty differentiating depression from normal grief or normal mood swings. It is very hard for most of us to tell when our depression has crossed over from normal discouragement related to failure, loss, or disappointment to a dysfunctional depression. Furthermore, the negative stigma associated with depression makes us feel embarrassed over having this condition, so we deny it to ourselves, claiming that there is nothing seriously wrong and that the sadness will pass with time.

Depression is not easy to identify even for professionals used to making this diagnosis. *Masked depression* (depression that is covered up by other behaviors or health conditions) is very common. Depression may be masked by self-medication with drugs or alcohol, self-treatment with gambling or sex, or physical symptoms that are misinterpreted as coming from medical causes.

On the other hand, weight loss from cancer or other medical conditions, reduced emotions due to Parkinson's disease, or reduced motivation seen in Alzheimer's disease, dementia, or mental conditions such as a personality disorder, anxiety disorder, or schizophrenia may first appear with symptoms that are similar to depression or may actually have depression as a complication. Discerning which came first is more of a challenge with depression than answering the old chicken-and-egg riddle.

If proper diagnosis of depression can be difficult for trained professionals, it is only reasonable that for a nonprofessional it would be much harder. This is why, as the saying goes in medicine, "He who treats himself has a fool for a doctor." If doctors are foolish to treat themselves, their families, or even their friends (because of denial that something might be wrong or the lack of objectivity another doctor might provide), then it is surely prudent to seek an objective professional opinion when the signs or symptoms of depression are evident.

In my case (DB), the first doctor to notice my depression and to offer help was someone I had known in New England but whom I visited after he moved to California. He discerned from my demeanor and my conversation that I was depressed, and he provided me with samples of one of the best antidepressant medications available at the time. I took that medication for nearly a year without seeing much progress, and the doctor had no way to monitor my progress because we lived on opposite sides of the country. It took some time before I finally got up the nerve to tell him, because we both were hoping that this medication would help restore my mental health, and I did not want to disappoint him with a negative report. Additionally, I knew almost nothing about such medications at that time, so I didn't realize that discovering the right medication in the right dosage for each patient is quite often a matter of trial and error.

So there I was in New Hampshire, taking medication that I wished I didn't need and that wasn't helping me. The realization that the latter was true came around daybreak one morning in early spring when I realized that I found the sound of singing birds outside extremely irritating. This shocked me enough to motivate me to tell the doctor what was going on. Immediately he prescribed a similar, but slightly different, medication at a higher dosage. Within a few days of beginning that medication, the mud-covered glasses were coming off and the singing of the birds started sounding good again. Such a dramatic change in such a short time with any of these specialized medicines is uncommon. I think in my case, the fact that I had been taking one medication for so long had set the stage for the second one's almost immediate effect.

I could have avoided months of anguish had I been wise enough, once my depression had been professionally diagnosed, to see someone locally who could monitor my progress. Like most depressed persons, however, I was blind to the degree of my depression until the birds woke me up to it.

Myth 7: Depression is just another word for grief.

Normal grief occurs when someone loses a close friend or family member (or even a favorite pet). In such circumstances it is normal to feel sad or down and to cry when one thinks about the departed loved one. Most people must work through certain stages of grieving in order to fully resolve their sense of loss. If this does not occur, most likely they will become depressed later . . . perhaps much later.

Such a delayed reaction often occurs in social contexts that reward saying the right things and doing the right things when a person is grieving, expecting that person to pretend the loss does not really hurt. Months, or possibly years, later when loneliness and sadness over the loss envelop this person and the natural process of grieving actually begins, he or she may be criticized by those who should have been encouraging and supportive through the entire process—encouraging the person to tell the truth and supporting him or her through the pain of facing that truth head-on.

Elisabeth Kubler-Ross, M.D., originally came up with the following five stages of grief based on her work with dying people and their families, as described in *On Death and Dying:*

Stages of Grief
- The first stage is *shock or denial.* You can't believe what has happened. You refuse the reality of it. It takes a while, sometimes a long while, for the full horror to seep in.
- The second stage, once you have fully grasped what has happened, is *anger or resentment.* Where someone has died from an illness, it is common for anger to be directed toward the medical entities involved. When someone dies in an accident— for example, as a result of driving too fast or while intoxicated— it is normal to feel some anger toward that person. If you believe a certain severe loss could have been prevented had God intervened, then it is only normal to feel resentful, even angry toward God (though such feelings are often suppressed or denied by believers because they think they are wrong). In both of the latter two situations, anger is often followed by a sense of

guilt, which can initiate a vicious downward cycle that leads inevitably to depression.

- The third stage is called *bargaining,* which involves trying to make a deal with God—"If only God would take this away, make it not so . . . , etc., then I will change my life, dedicate it to serving others, and so on."
- The fourth stage, *depression,* begins when the grieving person realizes that God cannot be manipulated by a let's-make-a-deal approach. The reality takes hold that the loved one has died or will die regardless of all that one may do or try to do. (These stages also describe the process of grief for a terminally ill person and his or her loved ones.) For those who cannot face such a reality, the force of the emotions involved may be directed toward themselves in the form of remorse or guilt. This can lead to an obsessive preoccupation with trying to answer questions such as "Am I being punished for something I did in the past?"
- The final stage is called *acceptance,* in which the grieving person decides to get on with life since nothing can be done to change what has happened. What many secular writers labeled as acceptance is, in reality, existential resignation—"I think I'll stop beating my head against this wall because the wall doesn't budge and my head just hurts." In our opinion, true resolution of grief is only possible in the context of faith. As the apostle Paul says, because we are not ignorant concerning the destinies of believers who now sleep in Jesus, we do not grieve in the same manner as those who are without hope.[12]

In our opinion, true resolution of grief is only possible in the context of faith.

The feelings associated with the depression of grief may come and go for a year or more, becoming more intense on birthdays, holidays, or anniversaries. For some losses that are particularly severe, this periodic sadness may last an entire lifetime.

Myth 8: Christians will be understanding and supportive.

"If somebody comes into my church," a famous preacher boasted, "and they look like they got up on the wrong side of the bed . . ." He paused for emphasis and momentarily affected the face and posture of a chronically depressed person. "Then I just want to go on down there and tell them to go back home and get up on the *right* side of the bed!"

Often the depressed of our day are nearly as marginalized, ostracized, and stigmatized as the lepers of Jesus' day.

A similar perspective is common in many evangelical churches today that may consider depression to be a cardinal sin because it violates one of the church's primary tenets—that Jesus wants us happy. Or to say it another way, depressed Christians are like lepers in a congregation convinced that Jesus wants us all to be healthy.

What Jesus really wants is for us to know true joy (versus happiness, which comes and goes). He also wants us to be whole. Often the depressed of our day are nearly as marginalized, ostracized, and stigmatized as the lepers of Jesus' day. It is high time that the stigma attached by many in the church to their brothers and sisters with depression be exchanged for the attitude the Lord had toward first century lepers, which was to reach out and touch them in loving-kindness when no one else would even go near them.

In her book *A Joy I'd Never Known*, Jan Dravecky honestly portrayed the spiritual shaming she experienced at the hands of her pastor and friends during her depression. After having taken Prozac for a few months, during which her true personality had returned, Jan asked her doctor to wean her from the medication partly because she couldn't shake the impression that having to take an antidepressant was a spiritual defeat. As a result, depression's fog slowly returned. About five months later, Jan attended church on a Sunday morning to hear a sermon obviously directed at her. "If you are depressed," the pastor asserted, "you don't need medication, you don't need counseling, you don't need to go running after everything the world has to offer. That will only open you up to the power of Satan and take you further and further into the realm of the Enemy. By turning away from the Word of God as your only source of truth, you invite, no, you welcome, the attack of the Enemy. No wonder you are depressed! You need to repent and sacrifice yourself at the base of the cross!"[13]

We could include more stories like Jan's, but we don't want to sound like we're indicting the church, since some churches are making an effort in this arena (and we hope more will do so). Yet the truth is that while we've heard many stories like Jan's, seldom have we heard of Christians making it their mission to reach out to the depressed among them, or better, to the depressed in their community at large. Without doubt, turning this particular myth on its head in Jesus' name would go far toward convincing observers in the community that his followers actually are willing to be like the one whose name they bear. Christians can do this by adopting Jesus' attitudes of gentleness, mercy, and kindness toward those who hurt—for "a bruised reed he will not break, and a

smoldering wick he will not snuff out" (Matt. 12:20; see also Isa. 42:3).
Pastors and other believers could show concerned compassion by leaving the ninety-nine sheep safely in the fold and going out to find and
rescue the one who is lost (see Luke 15:4–6).

Myth 9: Depression is a waste of time.

One popular Christian book actually says that depression is a waste of
time. Yet when you take a God's-eye view—remembering that he is not
in a hurry—you see something else. For the Scriptures are clear that God
is going somewhere in our lives, remaking us into the image of Christ.
How long this process takes or the methods required are secondary to
achieving the goal. Anything that is being remade experiences some
degree of distress, but the craftsman works with the end in mind. When
a woodcarver was asked how he made an Indian out of a log, he said, "I
just chip away everything that doesn't look like an Indian." Depression
is one tool (though not the only one) that God, the master craftsman,
employs to make us into people he can use.

The following quotations from people God has used very significantly should dispel the myth in question. Bible translator J. B. Phillips
wrote,

> It seems to me that, for the Christian anyway, the undoubted evil of
> this form of suffering can be turned into good by learning a deeper trust
> in the real and living God. It may be that we have relied too much upon
> the props of true and earthly friends. But in this painful experience we
> are stripped of our pride and pious imaginings. Temporarily at least we
> have no one who can understand what we are going through. We are
> alone in this bewildering world and our only hope is in God, not prob-
> ably the God who has satisfied us in past years or the God whom we
> imagined for our comfort, but the Spirit behind all creation. It is to
> know more deeply this real true God that we are permitted to go
> through the pains and humiliations of mental pain.[14]

The Roman Catholic mystic St. John of the Cross (1542–1591) says
in his masterpiece, *The Dark Night of the Soul*, that novices in the faith
take great pleasure and perhaps some pride in meditating on God and
fulfilling their obligations of service to him. St. John of the Cross believes
that such pleasure and pride (still common among people of faith today)
hinder God's purposes with the soul; specifically, that the soul will come
to a place of pure contemplation and union with God, who is love. In

God's purpose in allowing his children to experience the dark night of the soul is to rid them of the superficialities of their faith in order to draw them to a deeper knowledge of and dependence on him and only him.

other words, God's purpose in allowing his children to experience the dark night of the soul is to rid them of the superficialities of their faith in order to draw them to a deeper knowledge of and dependence on him and only him.

> Because the gold of their spirit is not yet purified and refined, they still think of God as little children, and speak of God as little children, and feel and experience God as little children, even as Saint Paul says (1 Corinthians 13.11), because they have not reached . . . the union of the soul with God. In the state of union, however, they will work great things in the spirit, even as grown men, and their works and faculties will then be Divine rather than human. . . .
>
> To this end God is pleased to strip them of this old man and clothe them with the new man, who is created according to God, as the Apostle says (Ephesians 4:24), in the newness of sense. He strips their faculties, affections and feelings, both spiritual and sensual, both outward and inward, leaving the understanding dark, the will dry, the memory empty, and the affections in the deepest affliction, bitterness, and constraint. . . .
>
> All this the Lord works in the soul by means of a pure and dark contemplation . . . [which is] the principal part of the purification of the soul.[15]

In other words, during the dark night of the soul, which seems to be a central part of depression for those who are spiritually inclined, we may feel blind, dry, empty, emotionless, and abandoned. These uncomfortable feelings are, however, not ends in themselves, or clinging to our faith by our fingernails would be just another exercise in futility. These feelings are a means to the end of the refinement of our faith and the primary way that God shows we who experience the "dark night" that he is all we need.

Though many modern Christians mouth the word *dependence,* in reality they only depend on God to do for them what they cannot do for themselves. As a result, God is more or less an addendum to their daily lives. Those who have journeyed with him into and out of depression *know* (experientially and not just theoretically) that they can only survive when God, in every present moment, is the first and only focus of their faith.

God has a purpose in all that he causes or allows. In other words, he is going somewhere in our lives. The question is: Are we willing to go there too—on his terms, not ours? Whatever it takes, even depression? Surely, the mere consideration of these questions is not a waste of time.

Their resolution is, for many, the pathway to purpose and fulfillment, even joy.

Myth 10: Depression arises from repressed anger.

Some popular Christian therapeutic approaches embrace Freud's theory of depression as "frozen rage," though they are far more directive about dealing with one's repressed resentments than Freudian therapists would be. Christian therapists who use this model of depression can be expected to probe a patient's memories for grudges from which the patient must repent, since holding grudges even temporarily is thought to be sinful. To support this view, they quote, "In your anger do not sin: Do not let the sun go down while you are still angry" (Eph. 4:26–27).

Depressed Christians may or may not experience this therapeutic approach. For believers, the main issue should not be whether this method works but whether its biblical foundations are valid. It is doubtful, for example, that the apostle Paul, who penned the passage above, intended it to say anything about the cause and cure of depression. The context of the passage is an extended comparison of the unconverted life with new life as a member of the body of Christ (Eph. 4:17–32). Here Paul is offering guidance to former pagans about *relationships within the church*. Believers, having put off the old self (including falsehood, anger, theft, unwholesome talk, bitterness, rage, brawling, slander, and malice), are to put on the new self with its new attitudes and actions. This new self is created to be like God in righteousness, holiness, kindness, compassion, and forgiveness—attitudes that are extended to other members of the church because in Christ God has forgiven us all equally.

"In your anger do not sin" is from Psalm 4, a psalm of David. The entire verse is: "In your anger do not sin; when you are on your beds, search your hearts and be silent" (Ps. 4:4). Though this is not a divine command, contained in this verse of poetry is a general principle that, when practiced, will produce a good spiritual result. That principle would go something like this: "When you lie down to go to sleep, search your heart, and if you find you are angry with someone, instead of attacking them verbally, choose to remain silent."

"Do not let the sun go down while you are still angry" is the apostle Paul's expansion of David's principle. Paul is speaking in generalities, since anger occurs as often at night as during the day. This, therefore, is a general principle for believers that, taken in context, means: "Be careful not

Anger is only one of many destructive attitudes that a depressed follower of Christ may need to put off.

to allow your angry feelings to give birth to sinful actions, thereby giving the devil a foothold [to impair your spiritual life]. Instead, without delay, forgive anyone whose actions have induced your anger, in view of the fact that God, for Christ's sake, has forgiven you."

We believe that when anger is a part of a clinically depressed Christian's constellation of unhealthful emotions, the Christian therapist should help that person to forgive the sources of his or her anger—whether living or dead, self or other—as a part of adopting a more constructive, mature Christian approach to living as an interdependent part of the body of Christ. However, anger is only one of many destructive attitudes (to self and others) that a depressed follower of Christ may need to put off. Focusing on the resolution of anger (repressed or otherwise) while ignoring a depressed person's uniquely unhealthy habits of thought or action will not facilitate true healing and may produce, in the patient and others, unnecessary psychic and spiritual pain.

If you as a patient are subjected to this approach and you believe you have transparently and forthrightly revealed your anger yet the counselor persists in trying to dredge up more, you should feel free to suggest to him or her that in relation to anger (or suppressed grudges), your conscience is clear before God because you are resting in the finished work of Christ and you would like to move on to other issues. Should your counselor remain in the grudge-hunting mode despite such a request, you need to find a different counselor, one willing to engage your depression in all its complexity.

Questions for Reflection

1. The myths and misconceptions we discussed in this chapter are listed below. Which of them do you think are typical of people in your church?
   - ☐ You're depressed because you want to be depressed.
   - ☐ You can beat depression with willpower.
   - ☐ You're depressed because of unconfessed sins.
   - ☐ If you're depressed, you're just feeling sorry for yourself.
   - ☐ Depressed believers have weak faith.
   - ☐ It's easy to tell when you are depressed.
   - ☐ Depression is just another word for grief.
   - ☐ Christians will be understanding and supportive.
   - ☐ Depression is a waste of time.
   - ☐ Depression arises from repressed anger.

2. Of these myths and misconceptions, which have you been most likely to accept in the past?

3. Which section contained information or a statement that you found surprising?

4. Which section contained information or a statement that you found encouraging?

5. Rephrase the list of myths and misconception into "Ten Truths about Depression."

6. If you agree that it might be possible to become addicted to depression and you've seen this in yourself or someone you care about, describe its effect.

7. If you have known someone who had a delayed grief reaction, recall how surprised you felt at the time. Should you encounter such a reaction again, what will you try to communicate to that person?

8. In terms of depression, where do you think God is going in your life? Record your answer in your journal.

9. Then ask yourself: *Do I want to go there too?* and record your answer to that question. If your answer is "yes," then ask yourself one more question: *Am I willing, whatever it takes?*

10. Compose a prayer that expresses these thoughts and record it in your journal. In a group setting, have all who wish to share their prayers do so, and then pray for one another.

PART 2

THERE
IS HELP

CHAPTER 5

Strategies and Pitfalls for Those Who Wish to Help Themselves

One day in the middle of winter, I (DB) went to get a haircut. The new hairdresser asked what I do for a living. "I edit a medical magazine and write books," I said.

"Really," she responded. "What kind of books do you write?"

I never know how to answer this precisely, so I said, "Mostly religious. I am a minister by training."

"That's interesting," she said. "What are you working on now?"

"A book on depression," I said, trying to find a way to help her keep her mind on her work. The next thing I knew, another hairdresser (unoccupied at the moment) had taken the seat next to me. She was doing her nails, and she kept working on them during the rest of the conversation, which was mainly between her and me.

"What do you think of Zoloft?" she asked.

"It's a good medication," I said.

"Really? Have you used it?"

"Yes."

"Doesn't work very fast, though, does it?"

"For most people it takes a couple of weeks at the right dose to feel a difference," I replied. "But in my case I had been taking Prozac for about a year, so I think that made a difference. I started feeling better in just a few days."

"They both work on serotonin, don't they?"

"Yes. They're selective serotonin reuptake inhibitors—SSRIs," I said, figuring that she probably knew what that meant too.

Taking charge of your health is a good idea, but you should only try to treat your own depression if it is very mild.

"How long does it take to disappear from your bloodstream?" she asked.

Wondering where she was headed, I said, "I'm not sure. But I think it might take a couple of weeks."

"So it would show up in a physical for the police force, wouldn't it?" she asked.

"I'm not sure that prescription drugs are an issue for police departments, but if they did screen for prescription drugs, it might show unless you waited long enough."

She seemed disappointed. "Well, what about St. John's Wort?" she continued. "Doesn't it have the same active ingredient as Prozac? How could they know if you were taking Prozac or St. John's Wort?"

"I doubt it's the same ingredient as in Prozac," I said (resolving to find out as soon as I got home). "I used St. John's Wort for awhile, but it didn't do anything for me."

"What about SAM-e?" my hairdresser asked. "A lot of people are using that."

"I tried that too," I said. "And it didn't do anything for me either."

The conversation continued for a while. I was impressed that both women were fairly well informed about various therapies for depression. Yet neither seemed very depressed. Perhaps they, like millions of people in the United States and Europe, are self-educated consumers who employ various over-the-counter, alternative remedies to counteract occasional mild depression or simply to elevate their mood.

Taking charge of your health is a good idea, in general. For the more you know about treatment options and the more aware you are of your overall health, the greater the likelihood that you will know whether you are doing okay without professional help or whether you need assistance. The bottom line in terms of this chapter's theme is that you should only try to treat yourself if you have very mild depression, not major depression.

Mild Depression

You are only mildly depressed if:

- You feel a bit discouraged or a little blue, perhaps bored.
- These feelings have been around for a few days or weeks and they tend to come and go.
- The feelings are tied to a specific situation or situations.
- You feel that you need a change (you're not happy about the way your life is going).
- You are hopeful about the future, but you're not enjoying life quite as much as you might.
- You're not having difficulty with sleep or your appetite.
- You're not losing or gaining significant weight.
- You've got fairly good energy, motivation, and interest in a variety of activities.
- Your ability to concentrate is not impaired.
- Your moods are not causing significant problems in your relationships (home and friends) or at work.

Six Self-Help Strategies to Counteract Mild Depression

If you search the internet for "depression self-help," you'll find more than 100,000 entries. Obviously a lot of people and/or organizations are anxious to help you help yourself. Their recommendations may range from the sublime to the ridiculous, but the most common recommendations include: meditation, self-hypnosis, goal-setting and time management, stress management, relaxation techniques, exercise, and support groups. The important thing to remember is that while those strategies and the ones we list below can help *anyone* feel better, they are not cures or replacements for professional help for anyone who is more than mildly depressed.

1. Enlist Constructive Friends

Christians are part of a worldwide body of believers. Because we share the same life-giving Spirit, who gives to believers spiritual gifts that are to be exercised in love for the common good, we are therefore mutually interdependent. We need others and they need us. Even when we feel weak, worthless, or unimportant, we still have a part to play in God's grand scheme of things.[1] When even mild depression clouds our spiritual vision and we feel afraid or ashamed or we want to hide, we remain no less interdependent. So it is not only acceptable but wise to seek help from others who will help us recapture the joy we've lost, reconnect with authentic faith, and refocus our vision to fulfill our sense of calling. Constructive friends like these may be rare, but they do exist.

By contrast, we're not obligated to continue with or cultivate friendships that have been (or may be) destructive. While it is true that we need others to hold us accountable to our pursuit of wholeness (see the covenant at the end of this chapter) relationships with judgmental people can heap guilt upon depressed people for not measuring up to certain human standards or expectations, when God may actually be pleased with our progress. While some observers may critique the speed of our recovery or the very fact that we struggle with depression, we are God's servants (not theirs), and the satisfaction of our true Master is our primary concern.[2]

People who are affected by mild depression need not critics but coaches[3]—wise and loving friends who will help them chart and maintain a course toward recovery. One very constructive function in this context is that a friend may keep the struggling person in touch with

Having at least one intimate friend who knows and loves us is a major component of mental and spiritual health.

Recreation can be re-creational.

reality, which is very hard to do when the only voice one listens to is his or her own. Without this assistance, even a mildly depressed person may become focused on a continual inner monologue that sounds something like this: "You might as well give up. How can you claim to be a Christian when your life is such a mess?" Although it is possible to learn how to counteract such negativity with positive self-talk without the help of a coach, this problem likely will intensify if the only voice responding is your own.

One way or another, we all need to know and embrace truth in our inner selves, allowing this truth to change our perspectives and inform our relationships. Whatever we call a person who is able to help in this way—coach, counselor, or friend—it is good to keep in mind that before there were psychiatrists, there were friends who took long walks together, listening, sharing, and caring. Having at least one intimate friend who knows and loves us is a major component of mental and spiritual health.

2. Engage in Healthful Activities

Regular exercise and maintaining a healthy diet will make you feel better physically and consequently will also improve your mental outlook. You can really capitalize on the values of walking, for instance, when you combine prayer or hymn singing with it, either alone or with others—as described in the book *Prayer Walk*.[4] Try listening to Bible tapes or inspirational speakers on cassette or CD while walking or running. These activities can accomplish both spiritual and physical goals. Engaging in more strenuous physical exercise such as running can release endorphins, a natural analgesic, in your brain, and this can also improve your mental outlook. However, if you're considering strenuous exercise, you should consult your doctor first.

For a long time, before my (HK) arthritis prevented this kind of activity, I would ride my stationary bicycle as I did my Bible reading. The exercise kept my mind alert so I could concentrate on the Scriptures, and the Scripture reading kept my mind occupied so I didn't think about the pain of exercise. At the end of forty-five minutes, I was feeling both physically and spiritually fit.

In my (DB) experience, time spent in the outdoors, especially in the mountains, is healing in itself. Often when I am hunting in the wilderness, I am not so much pursuing game as being pursued by God, whom poet Francis Thompson called "the hound of heaven." God speaks to me through the grandeur of the Rockies, the delicate beauty of tiny wildflowers, the delectability of wild mushrooms sautéed in butter, or the awesome power of an afternoon thunderstorm. There must be some endorphins involved, since a lot of the activity occurs at an elevation of about 10,000 feet, giving *hiking* (at least in this context) a unique cardiovascular meaning.

Through more than forty years of hunting, I've probably spent *years* in tree stands, waiting for deer or other game . . . but mainly enjoying the sun rising and the sun setting, as most of the natural world came alive around me in the morning and then retired with the sun later in the day. For some reason, being eyeball to eyeball with a surprised squirrel or confused chickadee helps put the right perspective on my worries. Although I can recall times afield when I struggled deeply with issues or decisions, I cannot recall many days spent outdoors when I returned to camp depressed. On the other hand, there have been many days of physical exhaustion combined with spiritual refreshment, which for me is recreational. Perhaps the most cleansing times occurred while wading northern New England streams, fishing for trout, but mostly letting the water wash my worries away.

3. Let Yourself Relax

God never intended for our lives to be all about work. Even he, when he had finished with the creation, entered the "Sabbath rest." You've heard the saying "All work and no play makes Jack a dull boy." Let's amend that statement in our context to say: "All work and no play makes Jack or Jill *depressed*."

Take time to enjoy activities with friends, take vacations with loved ones, and *regularly* get away from all stress for a period of time. You will not be able to totally eliminate stress from your life—no one can—but you can learn to manage it proactively instead of feeling like you are at its mercy. This management of time, energies, and resources may seem difficult, especially if you feel victimized by life in one way or another, but taking time to set goals can give you a new sense of mastery of your situation with all its problems. Two books on this subject that we highly recommend are *Margin* and *The Overload Syndrome* by Richard A. Swenson, M.D.[5]

Retreat centers operated by different Christian groups will allow you to spend a long weekend in the mountains or somewhere in nature where you can focus on reflection, scriptural study, prayer, and fellowship. These times can be enormously refreshing. You may think that you

All work and no play makes Jack or Jill depressed.

can't afford the luxury of such a retreat, but the truth may be that you cannot afford not to go.

Megan, a patient of mine (HK) who had struggled with depression for nearly a decade, found that her entire perspective on life changed during a weeklong retreat at a Christian center in the Appalachian Mountains. She was taking antidepressants and seeing a counselor, but she had done so for years with only partial relief of her symptoms. At the retreat, far away from the stresses of her work and family life, during one of the meditation sessions something inside of her suddenly clicked. She had a spiritual revelation about herself. This was followed almost immediately by a deep sense of peace. That peace continued for many months after returning to the real world. When things got crazy in her life, Megan would recall that experience and find the peace again. She found that attending the retreat two or three times a year (combined with continued therapy and antidepressants) helped to control her depression.

4. Volunteer

Helping those in need can counteract the boredom we sometimes feel, especially when our focus is entirely on our own pleasures or pains. Encouraging and supporting others who are struggling with life's problems can refocus our attention. When we love our fellow human beings as a service to God, joy begins to flow back into our lives.

Linda was struggling with self-esteem and guilt issues. Several months of psychotherapy and biblical counseling were not effective. Yet when she decided to volunteer one day per week at Agapé House, a home for wayward and neglected children, her depression began to lift. Soon she was volunteering three days a week and able to reduce the frequency of her physician visits from once or twice per month to once or twice per year. This activity gave her life a sense of meaning and purpose that helped to neutralize her feelings of inadequacy and regret. As she invested herself in the lives of these children, she took her eyes off herself. Rather than using all of her energies to psychologically beat herself up, she began to battle the negative forces that were destroying these young people's lives.

You might experience similar healing through volunteering, but it need not be at a children's home. Volunteering at a nursing home, a soup kitchen, or even an animal shelter might have a similar effect for you, though we believe your most satisfying volunteer experiences will involve helping other human beings.

5. Keep a Journal

Many depressed pilgrims have found that keeping a journal helps them see more clearly where they've been, where they are, and where they're headed. This activity can be a source of significant insight into the journey you're on. I (DB) have found that during the most difficult times of my life—when Jonathan was dying and after his death, and when Christopher was ill and I thought he was also dying—it was helpful to keep a journal for several reasons. Perhaps the most significant impact of the journal, over the long term, is that when I revisited those difficult times with the journal's help, I could recall how really desperate I had been. Without the journal to help me, I might easily have forgotten (or suppressed) the intensity of the pain along with the questions my suffering (and the suffering of my sons) raised as, like Job, I wondered about the meaning of it all.

Discovering answers to our deepest questions most often involves a drawn-out and painful process of reflection, grappling, and growth. A journal can help us recall this process and enable us to share any insights gained with others.

In a sense, keeping a journal helps us know *ourselves* better, since in those pages we describe what and who we care about—and other matters of the heart. We record our hopes, dreams, fears, successes, failures, and questions. In fact, over time a journal's pages may contain more questions than answers. Yet the questions themselves imply that we believe there are answers, even if we can't discern them now, because we believe our personal stories are part of a larger story, which has a beginning and an end, all woven together by a Storyteller who will one day make sense of it all.

A personal journal describes what and who we care about—and other matters of the heart.

6. Become Involved in a Prayer Group or Support Group

Whether alone or with others in a group setting, prayer can give great comfort, since this connects us personally with God and nurtures our relationship with him. That supernatural connection dispels loneliness and helps us put our problems in proper perspective. Active involvement in a prayer group can also connect us with others and make us aware that others are struggling in many areas of their lives.

Jane was depressed over the breakup of the relationship with the man whom she thought she would marry. As she isolated herself, she became more and more depressed, despite seeing a counselor regularly. One day a friend from church invited her to attend a prayer group that met once a week. The prayer group, comprised of eight people, opened with singing, and then a general prayer was said by the group leader. Each person, as he or she felt comfortable, updated the group on the situations they had prayed for during the previous meeting. If things weren't going so well, participants offered support and more prayer. When prayers were answered, everyone joined in praise and celebration. Toward the end, each person expressed prayer needs for the week following. Within a relatively short time, Jane went from being introverted and heavily weighed down by her problems to being one of the most active and helpful members of the group.

Other kinds of groups can also be helpful, including groups focused specifically on recovery from depression. Difficult as it may be to start attending such a group, when the group has a good leader and its program is constructive and practical, you will be amazed by the degree to which your issues and concerns are shared by others. As you listen and participate week by week, you may find that these fellow strugglers are the most understanding and supportive group of people you have ever known—and very likely you will come to count them among your best friends.

Eight Self-Help Pitfalls to Avoid

1. Most Alternative Therapies or Remedies

The most comprehensive Christian reference guide on alternative medicine, released in 2001, is *Alternative Medicine: The Christian Handbook* by Dónal O'Mathúna, Ph.D., and Walt Larimore, M.D.[6] This book would be worth buying if only for the excellent information in its sections "An Overview of Alternative and Conventional Medicine," "God, Health, Healing, and the Christian," and "Evaluating Alternative Medicine." The authors evaluate thirty-six therapies and fifty-six herbal remedies, vitamins, and dietary supplements.

Proponents have claimed effectiveness with depression for more than twenty of these therapies or remedies, including: aloe, Bach flower remedies, chromium, colonics, craniosacral therapy, DHEA, evening primrose, feverfew, ginkgo biloba, homeopathy, hypnosis, irridology, photo (light) therapy, magnet therapy, megavitamin therapy, Qigong, reflexology, Reiki, shamanism, St. John's Wort, Tai Chi, and Therapeutic Touch. While anecdotal evidence may exist in support of certain therapies or remedies mentioned here, it can be dangerous to combine some of them with prescription medication. So again, anyone consulting a physician for treatment of depression must be sure to mention any over-the-counter remedies he or she is using. In addition, some of these therapies can have detrimental spiritual effects, especially those that involve believers in trying to tap into or use forms of psychic or spiritual power that are not of God. If you are using or considering using alternative therapies for your depression, we urge you to consult *Alternative Medicine*.

Most alternative therapies are ineffective with major depression; some of them are physically or spiritually detrimental.

An extensive review of the scientific literature by Drs. O'Mathúna and Larimore prior to their book's release revealed trustworthy evidence supporting only St. John's Wort and photo [light] therapy as remedies that actually affect depression. Evening primrose oil, referred to in England as "The King's Cure-all," while effective in treating some ailments, had not been scientifically shown to alleviate depression. Although St. John's Wort may help with mild depression, a broad-based scientific study published in the *Journal of the American Medical Association* (10 April 2002) showed that while this remedy is safe and well tolerated, it is not effective for treatment of major depression.[7] Photo (light) therapy has been shown to be effective for the relief of seasonal affective disorder, which we mentioned earlier.

According to personal communication with Dr. Larimore, SAM-e was not included in the book because it was not one of the top one hundred herbs, vitamins, or supplements used in the United States, perhaps due to its higher cost. While studies have shown that some uses of SAM-e, especially intravenously and in conjunction with certain antidepressant medications, have been effective in the treatment of depression and other disorders, the problem of product quality remains for over-the-counter brands—the type most likely to be used for self-medication. In one independent evaluation of thirteen brands, nearly half did not pass testing. Among those not passing, the amount of SAM-e was, on average, less than half of the amount declared on the labels. For one product, the amount of SAM-e was below detectable levels (less than 5 percent of the labeled amount). Three of the products did not pass testing in part due to inaccurate labeling.

2. Avoiding the Pain through Overworking

When Adam was in the early stages of depression, which was related primarily to difficulties in his marriage, he threw himself into work at his florist shop. As long as he was at work, focused on his business and customers, he felt better. This activity took his mind off the problems he was having with his wife. Instead of dealing directly with his relational

"We work harder" is their motto, and they wonder how anyone could be critical of such an ethic.

problems, he spent longer and longer hours at work, finding excuses to stay late and spend time there on weekends. Eventually, the problems in his marriage worsened and his wife filed for divorce. This is when his depression deepened to the point that he sought professional help. While distraction may help to some extent in reducing the pain associated with conflict or loss, over the long term, avoiding a problem that needs to be resolved most often will only worsen the outcome.

Workaholism is an addiction for all who use work to shield themselves from experiencing the pain—psychic pain can be more painful than physical pain—of disappointments or depression. "We work harder" is their motto, and they wonder how anyone could be critical of such an ethic.

This self-treatment is common among people who are driven to achieve or to try to please someone—father, mother, spouse, church members, God, self, and so on. The problem with workaholism is that over time it has the opposite effect from what was hoped for. Instead of those around us being impressed with our efforts to please them, they may feel neglected, even alienated, because to the degree that we are immersed in work, we are not there for them. In other words, as we focus all our energies on secondary things, what matters most slips past us hour by hour, day by day.

God's view on this subject is represented in the story of Mary and Martha in Luke 10. Martha was rushing around, consumed with her preparations, while her sister, Mary, was content to sit at Jesus' feet and learn from him. When Martha complained, asking Jesus to tell Mary to help with the work, Jesus replied, "Martha, Martha, . . . you are worried and upset about many things, but only one thing is needed. Mary has chosen what is better, and it will not be taken away from her" (Luke 10:41–42).

3. Dulling the Pain with Alcohol or Drugs

For men, alcohol may be the substance most widely used to self-medicate for depression. As mentioned earlier, alcoholism is higher among men and depression is lower when compared with women. It is possible that the two are related—men would rather medicate with alcohol than talk about their problems with a psychotherapist or depend on an antidepressant medication to make them feel better.

This was true for me (DB). The following is adapted from an article I published in *New Man* magazine:

Gradually, like many men with broken hearts, I began to fill the hole in my heart with alcohol. But the more booze I poured into this hole, the deeper it got.

I struggled with this growing dependency, for I knew that only Jesus could satisfy my soul. But I didn't want to let go of the pain, for doing so would be to surrender: "God, you win."

I knew that beyond the wilderness of confusion and on the other side of the mountains of pain, with their valleys of depression, was joy, which was where God wanted to take me. But for years I insisted that if I was going to go there it would have to be on my own terms.

One day, when I was hiking near the Continental Divide in Colorado, I was struck by the awesome beauty of the golden aspens against the cobalt blue sky, and I began to thank God for making it that way. From this simple beginning, the rest came tumbling out. One by one, I laid down before God the things he brought to mind: my sadness, my bitterness, my career, my family. But when he brought up *the bottle* I realized that I couldn't imagine facing a day without it. That's when I knew I was in trouble.

I wish I could say the solution was simple, but anyone who has struggled with "demon rum" knows it doesn't let go without a fight. In fact, the struggle intensified over the next few months. The harder I tried to whip it in my own strength, the more I needed the bottle in order to fight the battle. And the more alcohol I poured into that hole in my heart, the deeper it became.

Finally, on Easter morning I was sitting in church thinking: *Either the Resurrection is real, or it's not. If it's not, then none of this matters, and I might as well go live in the mountains as a hermit with my dog and gun and a case of Old Grand-Dad and have some fun before I die, which won't be too long from now because I'll certainly drink myself into oblivion.*

But if the Resurrection is true, then the power that raised Jesus from the dead is available to me to live the life and fulfill the mission to which God has called me, part of which requires me to stop trying to fill my void with anything other than himself.

I wish I could say that I've never even wanted another drink. The fact is, the next month following that Easter day was the hardest month I have ever lived. Every day, nearly every minute, every cell in my body longed for a drink. But gradually, as my brain adjusted to seeing life without a haze, the desire diminished in intensity. Still, day by day, I must remind myself that the only way to fill the emptiness that I sometimes still feel is with a more intimate knowledge of God.[8]

> *If you try to fill the hole in your heart with substances, the hole will just get bigger.*

Alcohol itself is a depressant—not just of the mind but of the body too. So the net result of using alcohol to dull the pain of depression is

Treating the symptoms of depression instead of its causes will only compound the situation.

that depression intensifies. Using alcohol to dull the pain is bad enough; combining alcohol with drugs, whether street drugs or prescription drugs (or simply self-medicating with drugs) can be a recipe for disaster.

The most common abuses occur with central nervous system stimulants such as amphetamines, diet pills, or even caffeine pills. Some people self-medicate with antianxiety drugs such as Valium, Xanax, or Ativan. Some find relief by using painkillers such as Darvocet, Percodan, or Dilaudid. Others take over-the-counter sleeping pills (which usually contain an antihistamine like Benadryl that for older persons may affect memory or concentration) or prescription sleeping pills such as Ambien, Restoril, or Dalmane. Combined with alcohol, some of these can put you to sleep . . . permanently.

Many depressed persons are just trying to survive by using antianxiety drugs or sleeping pills. These may treat the anxiety and the insomnia of depression without treating the illness. It's like a person with a life-threatening pneumonia taking Tylenol for a fever without treating the underlying disease process that if unchecked could be fatal. These methods are tempting because they may produce a rapid relief of symptoms. The problem with treating just the symptoms of depression is that pretty soon you will have to increase the antianxiety medication or sleeping pills in order for them to work as the depression deepens. Also, a person may ultimately become dependent on the antianxiety drugs or sleeping pills, still without dealing with the real cause of their distress. So the net result is that the person's problems are compounded rather than relieved.

4. Substituting False Intimacy for the Real Thing

False Intimacy is the title of a book by Dr. Harry W. Schaumburg, who has a specialized ministry to those affected by pornography. Here is an excerpt from his group's web site, used by permission:

> Stealing a glance at a pornographic magazine. Surfing the Internet for sexual images. Finding more excitement outside of marriage than in it. Frequenting chat rooms on the Internet to find meaningful relationships. Soliciting a prostitute. What lies behind the struggle of sexual addiction?
>
> "Every person needs and longs for true intimacy," writes Dr. Schaumburg. "But, because of hurt and disillusionment encountered in close relationships, many people seek to fill their relational void through false connections—real or fantasized relationships that appear to provide the relief, acceptance, and fulfillment they long for. Pursu-

ing such connections regardless of the cost to one's reputation, health, security, marriage, and self-respect is characteristic of false intimacy."[9]

Anyone can fall prey to this method of self-treatment. Dr. Louis McBurney, who has now seen over 2,200 full-time Christian workers and spouses in his program at the Marble Retreat[10] in Marble, Colorado, describes a common scenario: "What we're seeing more commonly [than adultery] is an addictive, compulsive behavior toward pornography, particularly on the Internet, which seems like a safe place to go get some relief of your symptoms. Often, one of the things that goes with depression is an interruption of good sexual function, but in the context of pornography a guy doesn't have the same stress as he gets with his spouse, since he has no one to please but himself.

"When or if the spouse finds out about it, she needs to realize that this isn't about her [most, but not all with this problem are male]. Most spouses jump to the conclusion that if their husband is looking at naked women it's because he's not satisfied with her and her body. But what is going on has a lot more to do with how he feels about himself and his ability to cope with life, while remaining a potent person.

"Of course, sexual acting out with other women can be a big problem, too. That typically happens when a fellow is down, depressed, and he feels like everybody who comes through the door of his office heaps more criticism on him. All of a sudden this vivacious person comes in and gives him a lot of affirmation and tells him that she really appreciates him, how wonderful he is, and so forth. This support feels very good, and before long that relationship grows into something that's out of bounds. It doesn't usually begin about sex. It begins about his need for affirmation and acceptance, which just happens to come packaged in a female body."

The only real solution to this temptation is to deal with the underlying issue—depression, however it rears its ugly head. Relieving oneself via false intimacy only leads to addiction to false intimacy. When this happens, one's problems are only compounded, as the person will have to deal with the addiction first and then the depression that left him or her vulnerable in the first place.

5. Employing Other "Comfort" Solutions

Anything to which we turn to relieve our psychic pain quickly and without effort will bite us back, one way or another. Have you ever heard someone say, "The only real solution to this problem is a banana split (or

Relieving oneself via false intimacy only leads to addiction to false intimacy.

Psychosomatic symptoms are very real to people who have them, so telling them that "it's all in their head" will not usher in an instant cure.

a great steak, or chocolate cake, or some other delectable thing)"? Some people, when depressed, do not lose their appetites (which is more common) but become compulsive eaters. Eating, like drinking, is something they can do entirely on their own without depending on anyone else or going through the pain and effort of working through their problems.

Some, for the same reason, become compulsive spenders, taking all their credit cards to the max and then some in a vain effort to fill their own personal void with the acquisition of things. Secondary to this particular addiction may be the ego massage that comes from knowing that someone, somewhere will still grant you credit. In other words, someone somewhere still believes that you are worthy.

6. Developing a Variety of Physical Complaints

Before his crisis, Leonard was pretty healthy—weight was down; he slept well; he had no real chronic physical problems. Yet almost immediately after the crisis, Leonard began to wake up multiple times throughout the night. The tension he felt was unmanageable—especially in his upper back and neck. He was not able to relax, no matter how he tried. It struck him that if he did relax he would unwind like a spring. He started grinding his teeth during sleep, which was only relieved through the use of a splint he wore on his teeth at night. He developed a whole constellation of symptoms over time. Intuitively, he knew that all these symptoms came from the same source—unresolved stress that had become, over time, depression—he just didn't know what to do about them. The passage of time, despite the fable that it heals all wounds, only intensified Leonard's physical distress.

Symptoms like these are common to depression. They are called "psychosomatic" because their true cause is in the psyche rather than the body, even though the body is where the pain finds expression. Regardless of what the symptoms are called, they are very real to people who have them, so telling them that "it's all in their head" will not usher in an instant cure. (The truth is the symptoms are not all in their head. Depression is a whole-person disorder involving body, mind, spirit, and relationships.) However, psychosomatic symptoms can hide or mask the underlying issue of a person's increasing depression, and the longer this goes on, the deeper and more tenacious the depression will become. So getting treatment focused only on the symptoms (for example painkillers for the pain, muscle relaxants for back and neck, and sleeping pills for insomnia) will not usually solve the problem.

We don't mean to imply that all physical complaints are psychosomatic for those who are depressed. In fact, depression can itself be a secondary effect of certain other illnesses, so it is always a good thing to get a thorough physical exam and work-up if you begin to experience symptoms such as headache, backache, TMJ (Temporomandibular Joint Syndrome) pain, insomnia and/or constant fatigue, more than usual irritability, significant weight loss or gain, problems with memory, or confusion.[11] You need your physician to rule out other possible causes before anyone concludes that your complaints are depression-related.

Desperation for relief may drive anyone to pursue almost any avenue of relief.

7. Seeking and Embracing Easy Answers

Many of the pitfalls we've mentioned have in common the adoption of a relatively easy solution to a very complex problem. While this approach may be a typical human tendency, it is especially true for those who believe that depression is primarily a spiritual issue.

Sometimes depressed Christians seek a spiritual experience that will immediately eradicate their symptoms once and for all. Regardless of one's spiritual maturity, his or her level of desperation for relief may drive any person to pursue almost any avenue of relief. Some spiritual experiences may bring temporary emotional relief and release, and some may bring permanent healing.[12]

Should the symptoms return, as they often do, where can the depressed person turn? Family, friends, and church acquaintances, thinking the problem is finally resolved, would prefer to move on and not be dragged back into the pain of the supposedly "healed" person. In this scenario, he or she turns within, confused and guilty, and even more depressed than before since it is apparently true that he or she is not worthy of healing, health, and ultimately the wholeness that only God can provide. In truth, while God can and does sometimes instantaneously heal depression (and other diseases), healing of depression usually is a process occurring over time, just as the patient usually develops his or her depression over time.

The bottom line is to beware of *anyone* promoting *anything* as an easy fix to depression. People making such claims may be trying to sell you something.

8. Insisting You Can Help Yourself

This chapter's self-help strategies (and pitfalls to avoid) relate primarily to those who are mildly depressed. However, it is possible for a person's depression to be mild enough not to need the help of a physician or psychologist, yet still be severe enough that it is important to seek help from clergy or a noncertified Christian therapist.

More Severe Mild Depression

Mild depressions of a more severe nature involve symptoms such as these:

- You find yourself feeling discouraged, blue, or irritable rather often.
- You've noticed these feelings for several months now, but they are mild, not severe.
- The feelings seem to be related to one or more sources of stress in your life.
- The stress you're having is clearly related to the present, not to deep issues in the past.
- You may be feeling some guilt, but it is not severe and you're not obsessed with it.
- Your energy might be slightly down, and you may feel a bit drained.
- You can concentrate well and are thinking clearly.
- You're hopeful and motivated to feel better.
- There are no significant difficulties with sleep or appetite.
- Your moods are causing only minor problems in your family, relationships, or work.
- You still enjoy getting together with others and engaging in various enjoyable pursuits.

If this description fits better than the earlier one, then you will probably not be terribly successful in dealing with your depression on your own. Practicing this chapter's strategies while avoiding its pitfalls should help you, but if you insist on treating yourself, the process will probably take a considerable amount of time. You could avoid a lot of needless struggle and effort by seeking help from someone who is experienced in counseling people with problems like yours. He or she should be a mature adult who is emotionally and spiritually healthy and able to make you feel listened to, understood, and cared about.

Sometimes friends—and occasionally family members who are able to be objective enough—can fulfill this listening, understanding, and caring role. But most people find it easier to share intimate, potentially embarrassing details of their lives with someone whose only agenda is to help them sort it all out, resolve what needs to be resolved, and then move on constructively with living.

You may find that the above description fits your symptoms but you find yourself substituting words that are more intense. If you need stronger words than "discouraged, blue, or irritable," if you feel "exhausted most of the time" versus "a bit drained," if you feel "confused" more often than you can "concentrate well," or if you would really rather avoid social settings and only tolerate versus "enjoy" previously enjoyable pursuits, then your most effective help will come from one or more mental health professionals, as described in the next chapter.

Questions for Reflection

1. Do you think it is possible to take charge of your health? If so, what would this mean to you in relation to depression?

2. In your experience, do some people seem to feel obligated to critique the speed of a depressed person's recovery or to criticize the very fact that he or she struggles with depression in the first place? If so, how might you have responded when this happened? How do you plan to respond if it happens again?

3. Describe how you try to take care of yourself in terms of diet, sleep, and exercise. What could you do to improve in these areas? When would be a good time to begin?

4. If you were able to go on a personal retreat for a weekend, what setting would you prefer, and what would you do to use the time re-creationally (i.e., allowing the Lord to re-create or revive you in a spiritual sense)?

5. Does it raise your spirits or make you more depressed when you try to help someone else with their problems?

6. Consider the following quote from this chapter: "Keeping a journal helps us know ourselves better, since in those pages we describe what and who we care about—and other matters of the heart." If you are keeping a journal as you read and/or discuss this book, what have you noticed about yourself thus far that you hadn't noted before?

7. If you have participated in a prayer group or support group (or you are doing so as you study this book), describe in a sentence the value of this experience, and than share it in the group setting.

8. Review the "pitfalls to avoid." Which of these, if any, have you used, and what was the result in each case? What other pitfalls might you add to this list?

9. If you are mildly depressed, based on the symptoms cited, and you want to try to recover without involving a mental health professional or using medication, what is your plan?

10. If you think that accountability will help your process of recovery, list the name of a person or persons to whom you are willing to be accountable in this endeavor: _____

_____.

If you want to take this a step further, you might use the following covenant, or a variation of it, to reinforce your resolve (feel free to reproduce this in your own words in your journal, if you're keeping one):

Before God, I hereby state my intention to do the following to counteract my depression: _____

_____.

In this endeavor, I will not only be accountable to myself and to God, but I will also be accountable to: _____

_____. *Specifically, my accountability will take this form:* _____

_____

_____

Signed: _____ *Date:* _____

Recommended Reading

Issues Related to Depression

Backus, W., and M. Chapin. *Telling Yourself the Truth.* Minneapolis: Bethany House, 2000. For those with mild depression.

Biebel, David B. *How to Help a Heartbroken Friend.* Grand Rapids: Revell, 1993. Autographed copies available via e-mail at: *dbbv1@aol.com* or web site at: *www.hopecentral.us.*

———. *If God Is So Good, Why Do I Hurt So Bad?* Grand Rapids: Revell, 1995.

———. *Jonathan, You Left Too Soon.* Grand Rapids: Revell, 1997.

Bunyan, John. *The Pilgrim's Progress.* Nashville: Thomas Nelson, 1999.

Dravecky, Jan. *A Joy I'd Never Known.* Grand Rapids: Zondervan, 1996.

Graham, Ruth Bell. *Prodigals and Those Who Love Them.* Grand Rapids: Baker, 1999.

Koenig, Harold G. *The Healing Connection.* Nashville: Word, 2000.

———. *Purpose and Power in Retirement: New Opportunities for Meaning and Significance.* Philadelphia: Templeton Foundation, 2002. For the soon-to-be-retired person.

Kreeft, Peter. *Making Sense out of Suffering.* Ann Arbor: Servant, 1986.

Nouwen, Henri. *The Wounded Healer.* New York: Doubleday, 1979.

Schaefer, Edith. *Affliction: A Compassionate Look at the Reality of Pain and Suffering.* Old Tappan, N.J.: Revell, 1978.

Shields, C., and C. Ferrell. *Spiritual Survival Guide: How to Find God When You're Sick.* New York: Doubleday, 2001. For those with physical health problems.

Tada, Joni Eareckson, and Steve Estes. *When God Weeps: Why Our Sufferings Matter to the Almighty.* Grand Rapids: Zondervan, 1996.

Thurman, Debbie. *From Depression to Wholeness.* Monroe, Va.: Cedar House, 2000.

Walsh, Sheila. *Honestly.* Grand Rapids: Zondervan, 1996.

Winter, D. B. *Closer Than a Brother: Practicing the Presence of God.* Wheaton: Shaw, 1971.

CHAPTER 6

Mental Health Professionals
Who They Are and What They Do

"Up until just recently," Stephen wrote, "for as long as I can remember, I have awakened virtually every morning at three, four, or five o'clock with an ominous black cloud of anxiety, fear, and depression hanging over me. An almost constant thought was that death would be a welcome alternative to the thought of facing the rest of my life as it appeared before me. For a believer in Christ, this was simply not supposed to be the case, particularly for an associate pastor in a rapidly growing, charismatic church.

"My early morning pattern had been the same for about twenty-five years. I would stumble out of bed, fighting the flood of negative and condemning thoughts, and find my place in the familiar living room chair with my Bible open before me as I 'sat before the Lord.' There was simply no other way that I could face the day. It was as if the Scripture 'Man cannot live by bread alone, but by every word that proceeds out of the mouth of the Lord' was engraved on my heart and mind.

"Probably ninety-nine days out of a hundred, as I meditated in and prayed the Scriptures, within a matter of minutes I began to feel a peace that was simply indescribable. There would come an experiential knowing that he was and is everything that he says he is—my peace, my strength, yes, my very life. There would come an eternal perspective of hope and encouragement in the face of my fears regarding the day ahead of me as well as an assurance that the mistakes of the previous day were forgiven and forgotten. All I can say is that this unfailing presence of God was totally addictive. I could not, would not, had no desire to attempt to live without it.

"Often within an hour or two of leaving my time alone with God, gradually the negative thoughts would begin their relentless assault again, despite my intense efforts to ward them off. I tried with all of my strength to resist, but in every case the only way to continue the day with any sense of stability was to again spend time alone with God, opening the little New Testament that was always in my right back pocket. He was faithful to somehow always provide a few moments in the middle of the meeting or a break of some sort in my day when I could get alone with him, and once again he would come, driving back the darkness and impending doom.

"There were, however, seasons when the pressures of life, my tremendous feelings of inadequacy, and my inability to roll the cares of the people I loved off upon him would bring me to a place where I was unable to feel his presence. The black cloud of depression would become so oppressive that I was unable to function. During these horrible times, it was so clear to me that the obvious next step for me was to find something else to do—anything would be better than having to interact with people and talk about the Lord when he felt so distant. For some reason, however, my three best friends in life—my wife, my dad, and my senior pastor—refused to agree with me. Why, why could they not see that I was not the one for this position? Could they not see as clearly as I did that I was not really called, qualified, or capable of continuing?

"At perhaps my darkest moment in life, the Lord in his great faithfulness led me to Psalm 16:11, 'You will show me the path of life; In Your presence is fullness of joy; at Your right hand are pleasures forevermore' (NKJV).

"Could there possibly be a path out of this living hell? Could there be such an emotion as joy in my life? It didn't seem possible.

"Several days after this single ray of light appeared in the vast darkness, my dad convinced me to come see him and visit Dr. Koenig. With great reluctance I made the three-hour drive to Durham, dreading the thought of interacting with anyone. Why could Dad not understand that there was no hope of change in my life? Why couldn't he realize that I had always been this way, and that if I was in this state at age fifty-three, I would be this way forever?

"Dad asked me to promise that I would do two things, and he was very serious: I would agree to try medication, and I would be willing to receive counseling help. With great reluctance I agreed.

"Probably the most difficult step was the medication. During the first several weeks, things got even worse in terms of anxiety and sleeplessness, but eventually I began to feel somewhat better.

"How quickly I forgot the horror of 'the pit.' I discontinued the medication, and eventually the wave of depression overcame me again. My response to counseling was similar. As soon as I felt better, I discontinued the sessions with the counselor.

"After another year and a half of this roller-coaster existence, trying different medications with nothing really working well, I agreed to give it one more try at the request of my wife. After three weeks on a new medication, I experienced what I could not ever remember feeling. I woke up on Wednesday morning, March 27, and the cloud was gone! Since that amazing experience, I have had a few tough days, but nothing like the past. I sleep through the night, and I wake up in the morning without the cloud. I feel that if God never does anything else in my life, it would be okay. I have experienced a miracle.

"But he has done so much more! I now meet with a wonderful Christian counselor on a regular basis, and with his help I have gained an understanding of the performance orientation that has driven me all of my life. In my case, I believe that in order to come to a place of rest I never dreamed possible, I needed the medication to first quiet my mind so I could receive the insight and understanding God gave me through the counseling sessions.

"My love for the Word of God has not diminished in the least, but I can live without it being physically open before me throughout the day. I am beginning to experience as never before that he really does 'put [his] laws in [our] minds and write them on [our] hearts' (Heb. 8:10). For now that the barrage of negative thoughts has quieted and I can hear and heed his still, small voice as never before, I am experiencing what I was created to experience. I am able to love God with my heart, soul, strength, and *mind* as I never dreamed possible. I am also able to love others as God loves me (and as he loves them) because I am no longer consumed with thoughts of self—the great curse of depression.

"On the other hand, my depression has been a *blessing* because I can understand something of the pain and darkness in which others live. In some small way I have been there. As a result I can bring them, in prayer and faith, to God's throne of grace so that they, too, can find his marvelous, life-changing grace to help in their time of need."

Like Stephen, many believers stumble around in the dark, sometimes for years, trying to find a way through and beyond it. They may try some of the positive (or negative) methods of self-help discussed in the previous chapter. They believe that faith should banish the darkness of depression and fill their being with light. When it doesn't, they often

They did him the biggest favor of his life by insisting that he seek professional help.

begin to believe the lie that they are failures in God's eyes and not worthy to represent him in any way (or even call themselves Christians).

Fortunately for Stephen, those closest to him realized that his increasing despair was not an expression of his true self but was his depression talking. By that point, Stephen had been enshrouded in gloom for so long that his ability to perceive or accept anything positive had shriveled up like a flower in the darkness. So they did him the biggest favor of his life by insisting that he seek professional help.

For some people, agreeing to such a suggestion is very difficult. For a person whose ego has been ground to dust by months, perhaps years, of exposure to the ever-circling millstone of depression, the mere thought of being probed and analyzed by an as yet unknown person in an unknown setting using methods that are likewise unknown can evoke strong feelings of anxiety.

Our goal in this chapter is to alleviate some of this anxiety by providing an overview of the work of health care professionals, along with some suggestions about how to talk with them. For as your fellow human beings, they want to try to bring some light into your dark places so the wilting flowers can bloom again. Hard as it may be to attend that first session, doing so is far more constructive and responsible than continuing to hide or pretend, especially when those who care about us are unanimous that professional help is something that we need.

Who Mental Health Professionals Are

Believe it or not, anyone can call himself or herself a "psychotherapist" or a "therapist." No specific credentials are involved; no licensing is required. Certificates to hang on one's wall may be obtained via the internet. It is as essential for anyone seeking counseling to carefully inquire about the qualifications of a potential heart mender as it is to investigate the qualifications of a potential heart surgeon.

Counselors

Licensed or certified[1] *counselors* may be secular counselors, social workers, marriage and family therapists, Christian counselors, or pastoral counselors. All of these require meeting certain state or national requirements. Licensed counselors, particularly those who are members of the American Counseling Association,[2] have completed college or university and an additional year or two of training to obtain a master's degree in counseling from an accredited program.

Social workers (LCSW—Licensed Clinical Social Workers) also provide counseling. Social workers typically have a college degree plus two years of academic and clinical training culminating in a master's of social work degree (MSW). Besides learning to counsel, social workers also receive special training in case management and the use of social services and community resources. There are other variations of the Clinical Social Worker (CSW) designation, all of which require special training and licensure.

Marriage and family therapists (MFTs) are usually licensed (as of 2003, forty-two states required certification). They evaluate and treat emotional disorders and other health or behavioral problems within the context of the client's network of primary relationships (sometimes called a "family system"). MFTs have graduate training (a master's or doctorate) in marriage and family therapy followed by a period (usually two years) of supervised clinical experience. Many MFTs are members of the American Association of Marriage and Family Therapists.[3]

Christian counselors. Some people who are not licensed may call themselves "Christian counselors" because they are Christians who do counseling. If the counselor is not licensed, most likely he or she will not be a good choice for the treatment of major depression unless the counselor is working under the supervision of a physician or psychologist. Christian counselors who are licensed will have training similar to that of secular counselors. Some Christian counselors are members of the American Association of Christian Counselors.[4]

Pastoral counselors usually have a theological or pastoral degree in addition to a degree in counseling. In order to be certified by the American Association of Pastoral Counselors (AAPC),[5] a pastoral counselor must have graduated from college or university and a divinity school or seminary as well as have earned a master's or doctoral degree in counseling or psychology. Postseminary training must include at least 1,375 hours of supervised clinical experience involving individual, group, marital, and family therapy, plus 250 hours of direct approved supervision working in both crisis and long-term situations.

While many *clergy* provide counseling, their certification is often ordination to the ministry in general rather than counseling certification. Most will have completed seminary (three years of study after college). Some, however, will have attended Bible college directly after high school to obtain training for the ministry. The amount of training in counseling at seminaries and Bible colleges is highly variable, often minimal (compared to the training described for the AAPC, for example). As a result, many clergy do not have adequate theoretical or clinical training to recognize or treat major depression, though this has been slowly changing over the past few decades, at least at the seminary level. Even when they have adequate training and experience to recognize major depression, our view is that they should not attempt to function as the depressed person's only professional caregiver, since all persons with major depression need medical evaluation and treatment.

Psychologists

Most *psychologists* are mental health professionals who have completed college or university and between three and five years of postgraduate education to obtain an advanced degree in psychology (Ph.D., Psy.D., or Ed.D.). Many psychologists are members of the American Psychological Association, which helps to set educational and ethical standards.[6] Psychologists with only a master's degree may be licensed in some states, but they are not addressed as "doctor," since they have not earned that degree.

Christian psychologists attempt to integrate the strength of a person's faith together with secular counseling techniques to help their clients toward health and wholeness. Many are members of the Christian Association for Psychological Studies, a national association devoted to understanding the relationship between Christianity, counseling, and research, sponsoring education-related activities, and encouraging fellowship among Christians in psychology and related professions.[7]

Psychiatrists

Psychiatrists are medical doctors (M.D. or D.O.) who have completed college and medical school plus three years of psychiatry residency training. Those who have also passed a written and oral board examination are "board-certified" in psychiatry. Psychiatrists may be members of the American Psychiatric Association,[8] which serves the same purpose for psychiatrists as the American Psychological Association serves for psychologists.

Some *Christian psychiatrists* use biblical principles and religious faith together with secular psychotherapy and medications to treat patients. There is no national credentialing organization of Christian psychiatrists, though some may be members of the Association of Christian Therapists (ACT), a professional organization with strong Christian healing roots that arose out of the charismatic healing movement.[9] Their common bond is a commitment to Jesus Christ and openness to the gifts of the Holy Spirit, especially the gift of healing.

The Christian Medical and Dental Associations (CMDA)—a national organization with more than 17,000 members—has a psychiatry section. Patients can locate Christian doctors, including Christian psychiatrists, who are members of CMDA by accessing the organization's web site at *www.cmdahome.org,* then clicking on "Christian Doctor Search." If there are no Christian psychiatrists in your area, and your main concern is locating a physician who will focus primarily on helping you find the right medication and dosage, you should consider seeing a non-Christian psychiatrist for this purpose, combining his or her expertise with psychotherapy provided by a believer.

Medical doctors, though not considered an official part of the mental health system, also treat people for depression. Primary care physicians probably treat more depression today than do psychiatrists, since most people would rather consult their medical doctor than a psychiatrist. Also, because health insurers are encouraging medical doctors to treat depression rather than refer to psychiatrists, it is likely that this trend will continue to grow. Some medical doctors may have little interest or training in the treatment of depression, while others have a keen interest and skill in this regard. It is appropriate to ask your primary care physician about his or her interest and expertise in this arena and to request a referral if your doctor says (or you learn by experience) that he or she does not have adequate training or experience in the treatment of depression. Although many physicians in general practice are more or less up-to-date on the various antidepressant medications, their typical approach is to try one medication, then another, and another until a medication and dosage is found that relieves the patient's depression. This, in some cases, can take months, even years, leaving the physician frustrated and the patient disappointed, perhaps confused, and with less hope for relief than before. Although psychiatrists may also need to try several different medications until the right one (or combination) is found, they have more training and experience doing this, so the time necessary to find the medication that works for a given patient will likely be less.

Difficult as it may sound to do this, it is certainly better to make this change before launching into a trial-and-error approach to your treatment, which will surely be more painful for everyone involved in the long run than to receive treatment from a specialist right from the start.

Beware: Anyone can call himself or herself a "psychotherapist" or "therapist." No specific credentials are involved; no licensing is required.

What Mental Health Professionals Do

Counselors

Counselors use psychological and/or social methods to help relieve depression and stress. This is true for secular counselors, Christian counselors, and pastoral counselors (the latter two often incorporating spiritual methods as well).

You can expect a counselor to listen to your story, offer support and advice, and provide psychotherapy similar to what a psychologist would provide (though probably not as specific or as deep). You can expect the counselor to ask you about any suicidal thoughts and to monitor your progress and improvement. Any counselor (including a psychologist or psychiatrist) who feels that you are at risk for suicide is legally responsible to protect you—including arranging for commitment to a hospital.

A counselor may work in conjunction with a psychologist or psychiatrist, and some states require this for reimbursement under Medicaid or Medicare. Counselors typically do not do advanced psychotherapy (although some pastoral counselors do). Usually they do not offer psychological testing nor do they make diagnoses in the medical sense. They do not prescribe medications, and they do not treat patients who are suicidal without additional help.

Psychologists

Psychologists take your personal history and develop a diagnosis, although there is less emphasis on diagnosis and more emphasis on treatment, which typically involves some type of psychotherapy in which he or she may ask questions and listen carefully to your responses. Therapy provided is more than simply supportive counseling and is likely to involve techniques to address conflicts and hurts from the past. Examples of specific techniques used by psychologists include cognitive and behavioral therapy (or a combination of these), brief psychodynamic therapy, or interpersonal therapy. Therapies that involve cognitive processes and behavioral treatments are called reeducative therapies because they aim to reeducate patients in ways of thinking and behaving that will influence how they feel emotionally.[10]

Psychologists often administer comprehensive psychological tests to measure different areas of psychological, cognitive, and emotional functioning. The results help them decide what therapy to use and on which areas to focus. Ordinarily, psychologists do not prescribe medications, admit patients to the hospital, or administer electroconvulsive therapy (ECT)[11] or other biological or medical treatments. You can expect a psychologist to explain the therapy and testing that he or she chooses to administer and to monitor your response to this therapy. It is appropriate to ask for an estimate of how many sessions may be required before you should start feeling better.

Most people with significant depression need both counseling and medication.

Psychiatrists

Psychiatrists provide psychotherapy, prescribe medications, and when necessary admit people with serious depression or other emotional or mental difficulties to the hospital, where they also provide care. A psychiatrist may administer ECT to patients who are in the hospital. Today, psychiatrists are doing less psychotherapy and focusing more on treating with medications and other biological therapies like ECT. Depending on their interests, psychiatrists will vary widely in how much psychotherapy they provide and how much therapy is done by their associates who are counselors or psychologists. Most people with significant depression need both counseling and medication. A psychiatrist may see patients for a few minutes to check their response to the medications and to inquire about side effects. Then the same patients may see a counselor or psychologist in the same office to deal with psychological or social issues. Some psychiatrists may also refer patients for counseling in relation to spiritual issues.

If depression worsens despite treatment, a psychiatrist may adjust the medications or admit the patient to the hospital for more intensive therapy and to ensure the patient's safety. A psychiatrist should manage the care of all patients who have suicidal thoughts, delusional thoughts, or bipolar (manic-depressive) illness.[12]

Creating Effective Partnerships with Mental Health Professionals

Two things are certain: Your mental health professional needs to know your concerns, and you want him or her to understand what is important to you. If you use the following four principles, you and your provider of treatment should remain on the same page.

Four Important Principles

1. *Identify your main concerns before your appointment.* This is especially important prior to your initial visit. The first thing your provider of care will want to know is your chief complaint. This is what concerns you most. It is not up to you to provide a diagnosis of what is behind this concern; leave that to the professionals involved. Ask yourself: *If this person could do one thing for me, what would I request?* You may find it helpful to write things down beforehand. If you have more than one concern, prioritize them, but be aware that a list of three to five concerns may be all that can be handled in one visit. Next to each of your chief concerns, write the date that you first became aware of it. Describe in detail how it started, what its symptoms were, and what makes them better or worse. Be absolutely sure to tell your caregiver about any medicines you are taking, including prescription medications (which you should take with you) and any over-the-counter (alternative medicine) remedies, as some of these can have *serious* interactions with any new prescriptions this professional may wish to provide.[13]

2. *Speak up.* Even mental health professionals can't read minds. They may seem to be in a hurry, but they really do want to help you. Be sure your concerns, including your fears, are understood. You'll know this when the provider of care asks you questions about each concern you raise. Answer everything as completely and accurately as possible, as this will aid in diagnosis. If you have received *any* treatments in the past for things that still concern you, be sure to mention these specifically, since this may guide your caregiver toward a therapeutic plan that is tailor-made for you. (*Very important:* If you have ever experienced a manic episode, your physician needs to know this in order to properly manage your prescriptions.)

3. *Ask and answer questions.* Your professional caregiver will want to confirm the suspected diagnosis. A physician will most likely want to order laboratory and other tests. When you hear a term you don't understand, ask for an explanation. If you hear a diagnosis, repeat it back to the doctor or counselor. For example, you might say, "If I understand you correctly, you are saying . . ." Ask questions to clarify what the diagnosis means. For example, "What types of treatment are available?" "Please help me under-

stand how they work." "When should I expect improvement?" "What are the side effects, if any, and how should I let you know if I'm experiencing a negative one?"

If you forget to ask an important question during your visit, jot it down and ask it during your next visit. If a question is urgent, do not hesitate to contact the doctor's office immediately. Pleasant persistence pays off over time.

4. *Be sure to tell your mental health professional if you don't understand something.* For example, if a term is used that seems confusing, say, "I don't understand." Then, if a further explanation doesn't clarify things, you might ask for printed or audio resources to help you become more educated before your next visit. If no resources are available, ask for the scientific or common names for your diagnosis, and look it up at the library or on the internet. Your understanding and active participation in the treatment process will contribute to the process of your healing.[14]

Cooperate with Your Therapist

Sometimes after connecting with a professional (or team of professionals) who can really help, a person with depression may not cooperate fully. Often this can be classified psychologically. One response is *passive-aggression,* in which the person may be irritated or unhappy that he or she needs treatment. Since there seems to be no way around it, the passive-aggressive patient plays a "game" in which the goal is to punish those responsible (family, therapist, or both) by doing things or not doing things, depending on the situation, that might irritate or even anger the other(s). This result, to the depressed mind, seems to even the score at least a little, even if the whole thing is not consciously motivated.

Another possible dynamic is called an *approach-avoidance* conflict. In this case the patient knows that what is being offered is really in his or her best interests, but the anxiety or psychic pain of having to attend counseling sessions, or lowered self-esteem because medication is necessary, may produce all manner of rationalization or other avoidance activity:

"I really don't need this."

"I don't have time for this."

"We can't afford this."

"I'm going to be late again."

Any professional provider of treatment who feels that you are at risk for suicide is legally responsible to protect you—including arranging for commitment to the hospital.

"I can't make it this week."

"I don't feel well enough to go out."

I (HK) once had a Christian patient who would cancel appointments and refuse to take his medications. He didn't like having to see a psychiatrist and didn't want to be dependent on medication, as having to take medication made him feel less of a man. Consequently, his wife and two children went through untold suffering as they experienced day-by-day the consequences of this patient's depression. The patient was irritable, and nothing the wife or children did seemed to satisfy him. He was socially withdrawn and would not go out to social events with his wife, who was feeling increasingly socially isolated. He was not as emotionally available to his wife, had difficulty displaying affection towards her, and was completely disinterested in sex. He didn't have sufficient energy to play with his young children, who were desperate for affection from their dad. He was also not doing well at work, which placed his family under financial anxiety because they feared he would lose his job. To say it plainly, this patient's pride was causing unnecessary suffering for his family. Had he kept his clinic appointments, taken his medication, and made efforts in psychotherapy necessary to help change his outlook and behavior, most likely he would have spared his family a lot of needless grief and worry.

As his psychiatrist, I also felt frustrated. Eventually I decided to contact the patient's brother and wife to encourage them to place pressure on the patient to either get therapy or suffer significant consequences. One of those consequences was that the wife might temporarily pack up the kids and move in with her mother. Another consequence, if the depression worsened and the patient's safety became an issue, is that she might fill out commitment papers at the magistrate's office to have him taken, against his will, to a psychiatrist for evaluation and possible hospital admission.

Drastic measures like these are sometimes necessary to shock a patient into realizing how important it is that he or she not only seek treatment but fully cooperate with it. There are many things family members can do short of deserting or committing the patient, but sometimes the possibility that such things may happen will motivate the patient to be more responsible about following a treatment plan to which he or she has agreed. (See chapter 11 for more ideas and strategies related to how friends and family can help.)

Questions for Reflection

1. In terms of delaying or avoiding treatment, which of the following might be a factor for you if you were depressed?
   - ☐ denial that depression has happened to me
   - ☐ guilt that I am failing God
   - ☐ belief that taking medication for depression is unspiritual
   - ☐ concern that I am not relying entirely on God to get me through my problem
   - ☐ shame that I am failing my church, family, and friends
   - ☐ worry that others will think I am weak or worthless
   - ☐ fear of my secrets being uncovered
   - ☐ belief that I can handle this myself
   - ☐ lack of information about the nature of depression and the treatments available
   - ☐ anxiety that antidepressants will turn me into a zombie

2. What might help you get beyond this obstacle?

3. Which of these factors are affecting someone you love who is depressed and whom you would very much like to help?

4. What creative ideas occur to you in terms of helping your loved one past this obstacle?

5. Would you like to have Stephen on the pastoral staff of your church? If so, why? If not, why not?

6. Were you surprised to discover the wide variation among professionals who may be available to help with depression?

7. Would you want to be treated by an unlicensed/uncertified counselor or therapist? Explain your answer.

8. How would you discover the credentials of a mental health professional under consideration to provide treatment for you or your loved one?

9. Which factors related to a professional's credentials would be most important to you?
   - ☐ academic education
   - ☐ Bible school
   - ☐ college

☐ master's degree (including seminary)
☐ doctorate
☐ clinical experience
☐ spiritual maturity
☐ personal experience with depression
☐ ability to prescribe medication and/or other medical treatments
☐ openness to a multidisciplinary treatment approach
☐ biblical counselor (uses Bible texts and principles exclusively)
☐ integrative counselor (matches method to each individual)
☐ other:

10. Of the professionals listed in this chapter, which (or which combination) do you think would be most helpful to you or a person known to you who is clinically depressed?

11. As you consider creating an effective partnership with a mental health professional, what do you imagine to be the easiest and most difficult topics to bring up?

12. Explain why you agree or disagree with the following statement from this chapter: "If there are no Christian psychiatrists in your area, and your main concern is locating a physician who will focus primarily on helping you find the right medication and dosage, you should consider seeing a non-Christian psychiatrist for this purpose, combining his or her expertise with psychotherapy provided by a believer."

Concerns and Questions

Notes to Discuss with My Professional Treatment Provider

Suggestion: you might copy this, fill it out, and take it with you to each appointment.

My main concerns

Concern 1:

Approximate date I became aware of it: _____

History and symptoms:

It is better or worse when:

Concern 2:

Approximate date I became aware of it: _____

History and symptoms:

It is better or worse when:

Concern 3:

Approximate date I became aware of it: _____

History and symptoms: It is better or worse when:

Concern 4:

Approximate date I became aware of it: _____

History and symptoms: It is better or worse when:

Concern 5:

Approximate date I became aware of it: _____

History and symptoms: It is better or worse when:

My prioritized list of five concerns

1. _____

Treatments, medications, or over-the-counter remedies:

2. _____

Treatments, medications, or over-the-counter remedies:

3. _____

Treatments, medications, or over-the-counter remedies:

4. _____

Treatments, medications, or over-the-counter remedies:

5. _____

Treatments, medications, or over-the-counter remedies:

Questions I want to be sure to ask

1. _____
_____

2. _____
_____

3. _____
_____

4. _____
_____

5. _____
_____

What my professional caregiver said

1. _____
   _____

2. _____
   _____

3. _____
   _____

4. _____
   _____

5. _____
   _____

What my professional caregiver would like more information about

1. _____
   _____

2. _____
   _____

3. _____
   _____

4. _____
   _____

5. _____
   _____

CHAPTER 7

Counseling Models and Methods

Just as depression has many faces, counseling for depression has many forms. The method used by a particular counselor will reflect the counselor's training and experience as well as his or her understanding of human nature. If the counselor believes you need retraining in how you behave, the counselor will try to reinforce productive behavior (behavior that will alleviate depression) or to extinguish unproductive behavior (behavior that increases depression). If the therapist believes that repressed anger causes most of your depression, he or she is going to try to help you bring those repressed sources of anger to the surface so you can resolve them. If the therapist believes that religion is a cause for depression, you can expect to be urged to view faith in a different way.

The good news is that despite the wide variety of approaches to counseling, for milder forms of depression, psychotherapy (i.e., counseling or talk therapy) may be as effective as treatment with antidepressant medication alone or psychotherapy and antidepressants combined.[1] A variety of psychotherapies have been shown to relieve depression. There are perhaps a dozen competing models of depression, producing many different treatment approaches. These include cognitive, behavioral, cognitive-behavioral, interpersonal, marital (couples or family), group, and insight-oriented (psychodynamic) psychotherapies, including psychoanalysis.[2] There are also a number of less commonly used forms of psychotherapy such as reality therapy, gestalt therapy, transactional analysis, hypnotherapy, and art, dance, and music therapy. We will limit our discussion to the more common types of psychotherapy, while presenting a few hypothetical counseling sessions to give you an idea of what to expect from sessions using those therapies.[3]

Counseling Models and Methods	
Cognitive	Transforms false, maladaptive ways of thinking into adaptive, truth-based thinking.
Behavioral	Identifies behaviors that tend to maintain depression and then reduce or eliminate such behaviors.
Cognitive-behavioral	Counteracts maladaptive patterns of thinking and reinforces constructive behaviors.
Interpersonal	Teaches healthier patterns of relating to others.
Marital (couples or family)	Expects participation and shared responsibility of all parties in a marriage- or family-related conflict.
Group	Uses a variety of methods to teach new skills and provide understanding of the causes of depression in a group of people with similar problems.
Insight-oriented psychodynamic	Identifies internal conflicts and psychological defenses, providing insight into their causes.
Psychoanalysis	Helps patient uncover unconscious motivations and repressed memories and become aware of how these affect feelings and behavior.

Cognitive Therapy

Cognitive therapy involves learning to think in a way that is positive, optimistic, and reality-based. Depression can result from habits of negative thinking that magnify difficulties and barriers while minimizing positives about oneself, others, or situations. An unresolved question is whether negative, pessimistic thinking leads to depression or whether depression leads to negative, pessimistic thinking. Whichever is true, studies have shown that people can be trained to think in a positive manner and this will result in a lessening of depression, sadness, and suffering. Cognitive therapy attempts to transform false, maladaptive ways of thinking into adaptive, truth-based thinking.

Maladaptive ways of thinking include all-or-none thinking, selective abstraction, overgeneralization, personalization, and catastrophic thinking. *All-or-none thinking* is a tendency to think about situations as either black or white rather than in shades of gray, which is the way life usually is. For example, when considering one's abilities, a person might think: *I have no gifts or talents that are worthwhile,* or *I will never be able to play the guitar like so and so.* At another time, the same person may say, "I am the best piano player in the world," or, "I never make mistakes at my job." People who think this way may switch from one extreme to the other as the result of a single failure or a single success. There is an inability to see that oneself, other people, and most situations are usually highly complex, with both positive and negative aspects.

Selective abstraction involves focusing on the negative aspects of a situation while completely ignoring the positives. For example, a person who thinks this way might say, "I got a C on my report card. I am a bad student," while completely ignoring the three A's and two B's.

Overgeneralization is a tendency to draw broad conclusions based on a single event or limited amount of information. For example, "My friend Alice didn't call me last night. She must not like me anymore." Or after a single failed relationship, a person may conclude, "No one will ever love me again," or, "I will never find a compatible partner."

Personalization is a tendency to relate events to the self even when there is little evidence to suggest a connection. For example, a person sees two friends laughing and glancing his way. He concludes that they are laughing at the way he is dressed (when in fact the friends are laughing about something entirely different and just happened to glance his way).

Catastrophic thinking is excessively pessimistic thoughts about life. For instance:

"My situation is intolerable."

"I can't stand this emotional pain any longer."

"No one suffers like I do."

"This anxiety is out of my control."

"This depression is destroying my life."

"I can't live life feeling this way."

"My depression will never get any better."

Negative thoughts like these, often not based in reality, lead to painful emotions, fear, and suffering. Cognitive therapy helps people recognize these thoughts and their relationship to emotions and to consciously counteract negative thoughts with healthy, reality-based positive thinking. Cognitive therapy usually consists of eight to ten sessions,

*Cognitive therapy helps
people recognize and
counteract their negative
thinking habits with
positive patterns of
thought.*

though some health insurance plans may not cover that many sessions per year.

One reason we've covered cognitive therapy so extensively here is that it is becoming the talk therapy of choice, according to a Washington Post article: "Cognitive psychotherapy is the fastest growing and most rigorously studied kind of talk therapy, the subject of at least 325 clinical trials evaluating its efficacy in treating everything from depression to schizophrenia. For reasons both economic and cultural, it has begun to unseat neo-Freudian psychodynamic therapy as the dominant [psychotherapeutic] form of treatment in private and institutional practices around the country. For better or worse, cognitive therapy is fast becoming what people mean when they say they are 'getting therapy.'"[4]

SESSION

THERAPIST: *(male)* How are things going?

CLIENT: *(male)* There was a typo in my quarterly report. I put "your" instead of "you're." But I noticed it too late to correct it. When I gave that report to my boss, I just stood there waiting to be fired.

THERAPIST: Did he notice it?

CLIENT: Don't know. He didn't mention it . . . though I saw his lip twitch once while he was reading. The whole time I was in his office, all I could think about was that typo. I was so anxious I couldn't concentrate on what he said about my area's increased sales and that being remarkable given the current state of the economy. The rest was drowned out by a voice inside my head telling me how stupid I was not to have proofed the report one more time. When I went home after work, I couldn't eat. When I went to bed, I mulled it over for hours. By the time I fell asleep, I had myself convinced that he was just humoring me and that any day the pink slip will be on my desk when I get to work. I hardly slept at all. Every night since has been the same.

THERAPIST: Suppose you talked back.

CLIENT: To my boss? In situations like that I get so nervous that my main concern is trying not to faint.

THERAPIST: I meant talk back to the voice in side your head. Not out loud, of course. Nobody but you can hear what it's saying.

CLIENT: But it's the truth. I should have proofed it another time.

THERAPIST: How many times had you proofed it already?

CLIENT: At least five. Why I didn't see it until it was too late, I'll never know.

THERAPIST: You could tell your inner voice that you did your best.

CLIENT: But my best wasn't good enough.

THERAPIST: Now *I'm* hearing your inner voice. Since evidently your best was more than good enough for your boss, let's consider the untruth you just told yourself. How about saying, instead, "I gave it my best effort. That's all anyone can ask or expect of me." Repeat that after me.

CLIENT: But . . . I don't know if I believe that. I mean, it's not all I expect of myself. I expect myself to get it right.

THERAPIST: I understand, but I would like to hear you say what I said.

CLIENT: I gave it my best effort. That's all anyone can ask or expect of me.

THERAPIST: Good. Here's an assignment. At the beginning of each day, say to yourself: "Today I will give it my best shot. That's all anyone can ask or expect of me."

CLIENT: I suppose I can try that.

THERAPIST: There's a mirror on the wall over there. Just for practice, go over and look yourself in the eye and say, "Today I will give it my best shot. That's all anyone can ask or expect of me." *(After client does this, therapist adds):* In addition, at the end of each day I want you to say to yourself, "Today I gave it my best shot. That's all anyone can ask or expect of me." Say these things to yourself every day from now until I see you again, and we'll talk about the next step then.

Behavioral Therapy

Behavioral therapy attempts to identify behaviors that tend to maintain depression, and then reduce or eliminate such behaviors. Certain depressive behaviors (irritability, social withdrawal, etc.) tend to push people away and reduce pleasure and positive interactions with others. Other depressive behaviors (reduced initiative, unhappy or sad disposition) tend to elicit sympathetic and caring behaviors from others, which tend to reinforce depressive behaviors. In behavioral therapy, persons learn to identify depression-generating behaviors, acquire new social skills that will increase their positive interactions with others, learn problem-solving skills to increase successful interactions with the environment, and learn to structure time to increase pleasurable activities.

SESSION

THERAPIST: *(female)* So how was this week, on a scale of one to ten?

CLIENT: *(female executive of a nonprofit corporation)* About a two. I couldn't face the board meeting the other night.

THERAPIST: What's the problem?

CLIENT: Well, they seem to think I should be able to carry on as if happy thoughts and a pinch of pixie dust will make their Tinkerbell fly again. I mean, my husband walked out on me! And I was in Africa at the time, doing their business! It really ticks me off.

THERAPIST: It sounds like you think the board members are your adversaries.

CLIENT: Well, they're not *all* my adversaries. A few—actually a small majority, two women and one man—are on my side . . . sympathetic, understanding. They seemed satisfied that I showed up at all.

THERAPIST: And the others?

CLIENT: The others think I can be replaced—like getting a new wife, I suppose—even though I've taken the organization from nothing to where it is in just nine years. One of them even made a motion that I keep a record of all my business activities for the next month so they could know how I'm spending my time.

THERAPIST: Did the motion pass?

CLIENT: No. They tabled it after I clearly said that I was not willing to subject my work to that kind of intrusion. I think the guy who made the motion knows I've missed some appointments lately, and donations are down. Or maybe he was ticked because I arrived late . . . again.

THERAPIST: How late?

CLIENT: Not more than an hour. I didn't *plan* to be late. I started getting dressed with plenty of time to spare. But the closer the hour got, the slower I seemed to move. It's like my whole self went into slow motion.

THERAPIST: Have you considered going early?

CLIENT: That would be like showing up early for a root canal.

THERAPIST: If you were the first one there, you could greet them one by one as they arrive. There's no way around attending board meetings when you are the organization's CEO. You don't have to like it. But the way you're handling it now is alienating people *and* making you more depressed. Perhaps if you change your approach, other things will change too.

CLIENT: I could try it. I can't go on like this, that's for sure.

Cognitive-Behavioral Therapy

Cognitive therapy is often combined with behavioral therapy to counteract maladaptive thought patterns and engage the person in pleasurable activities and experiences that provide a sense of accomplishment and success in interactions with others. Thinking tends to influence behavior (for example, thinking good thoughts about others promotes positive behavior toward them), and behavior tends to influence thinking (for example, smiling at others promotes positive thoughts about them—and usually positive responses from them). Addressing both thoughts and behaviors, then, tends to be mutually reinforcing.

Cognitive-behavioral therapy counteracts maladaptive patterns and reinforces constructive behaviors.

Interpersonal Psychotherapy

This form of therapy focuses on a person's relationships and interactions, which are often a source of depression, sadness, and a sense of failure. The therapist explores and seeks to understand the positive and negative aspects of the client's interpersonal functioning. For example, if a person is coping with the death of a loved one, therapy might focus on helping the person left behind to establish a different identity (from that of a grieving spouse, for example, to a functioning single individual). Or the focus might be on correcting long-standing destructive patterns of social interactions. Studies have shown that learning new, healthier patterns of relating is often quite successful in relieving depression.

SESSION

THERAPIST: *(male)* You seem more down than usual today.

CLIENT: *(male nurse)* I can't help it. Someone put a note in my jacket pocket at the hospital last night. It said, "Isn't it time to move on?"

THERAPIST: What do you think it meant?

CLIENT: Well, I'm quite sure it was from Claudia, the head nurse. And it meant that if I continue letting my sadness spill over in a patient setting, I'm going to be looking for employment elsewhere.

THERAPIST: Perhaps there's a play on words here and she'd like to see you move on with your life . . . past your grief. How would you characterize your relationship with Claudia before Ron died?

CLIENT: Fine, as far as I was concerned. She seemed to respect my work and to appreciate my sense of humor.

THERAPIST: So maybe the note wasn't a threat but her way of trying to help you.

CLIENT: Am I supposed to turn off my feelings just because I'm at work? I mean my college roommate—my best friend—just died of AIDS. I haven't even told my parents yet. Claudia is the only person who knows what has me down. You'd think she, of all people, would cut me some slack.

Interpersonal psychotherapy focuses on interactions that may be sources of depression, sadness, and a sense of failure.

THERAPIST: It may not seem fair, but people do have expectations of professionals. At work you're in constant contact with sick people, many of whom are discouraged. Ordinarily, I'm sure you wouldn't want to drag them down further, would you?

CLIENT: That's true. I mean, I used to be able to find something cheerful to say. But now, especially if a patient's really sick, all I see is Ronnie.

THERAPIST: It sounds like you really cared about him.

CLIENT: *(nods)*

THERAPIST: And if you had been able to provide his care when he was dying, you would have not only nursed him well but you would have tried to cheer him up too.

CLIENT: *(nods again)*

THERAPIST: Is it possible, then, that when you see Ronnie in the form of a sick patient, you could care for that person as you would have cared for him . . . including trying to cheer up the patient? That way you wouldn't be denying your feelings but using them to help someone else.

CLIENT: I suppose I could try.

THERAPIST: Next time, I'll be interested to hear how it went.

Marital (Couples or Family) Therapy

Depression may result from chronic conflict in the home that leaves emotional needs unmet. One or both of the spouses may feel deprived of love, companionship, or similar needs. Depression can have a devastating effect on a marital relationship, especially when the depressed spouse is socially withdrawn, is irritable, or lacks initiative. When *both* spouses are depressed, their need for compassionate support is immense and immediate.

When there are children in the home, they usually internalize the pain of one or both of their parents; therefore, they often need support as well. Sometimes this dynamic is clear; for example, when the child of a parent or parents with depression suddenly begins to strike out at others or becomes a discipline problem at school. Often, however, the impact on a child is subtler, as when he or she becomes withdrawn or depressed. Over the past few decades a new approach has been developed, called "family systems theory,"[5] which seeks to treat each individual (couple or family) as a part of a system or network of relationships. When one part suffers, all suffer. When one is well, all are well. This is not only consistent with our biopsychosociospiritual model but also (in the case of Christian families) consistent with the apostle Paul's message about how all parts of the body need each other, and are therefore interdependent (see 1 Cor. 12:12–16).

Marital therapy is important for any depressed person who reports a troubled marriage. This usually involves both partners receiving therapy together, but on occasion they will meet individually with the therapist. The success of marital therapy depends heavily on joint participation and shared responsibility both for the conflicts that have arisen and in taking steps to resolve them. Even when a depressed spouse refuses to participate, the other spouse may benefit from therapy aimed at learning to cope with the depressed partner, which should help the spouse receiving counseling provide healthier support for the other.

When children are involved or are the reputed cause of family distress, the therapist can often identify clues that will help develop interventions by observing interactions between family members during joint sessions (or occasionally in the home setting). Family counseling usually involves the entire family meeting together with the therapist, though the therapist may choose to meet with individual family members alone from time to time.

SESSION

THERAPIST: *(female social worker)* How are you . . . both of you?

JUDY: Surviving, barely.

JIM: *(who recently lost his job)* More than surviving, with your help, thanks. I've been writing about losing my job. Just scattered thoughts for now, but maybe someday it will become a book.

THERAPIST: Judy, how do you feel about Jim's writing project?

JUDY: *(shrugs)* If he feels he has to do it, then I'm not going to stop him. But I wish he'd concentrate on finding another job. I hate having to tell Heather, that's our thirteen-year-old, that she can't go to a school function, or whatever, because we just can't afford it.

JIM: Well, maybe this will give her a little better appreciation of how we've sacrificed in the past so she could have everything her little heart desired!

JUDY: You have *no idea* how this has affected her. Her friends don't even bother to call any more; they're sick of hearing she can't go because we can't afford it. Sometimes I hear her crying in her room at night.

THERAPIST: I'd like to talk with Heather sometime soon, just to get her perspective on this. And after that, perhaps we could all participate in a session just to be sure that everybody understands every-body.

JUDY: That would be a good idea.

JIM: I don't see why we have to drag Heather into this, but if you insist. . . .

THERAPIST: Since your whole family system of relationships is affected by whatever happens, from events to psychological distress, it is best when everyone can participate in the healing process too.

JIM: Okay. But adding Heather's gripes to all the rest won't help me find a new job.

THERAPIST: How about a progress report?

JIM: Frankly, the job hunting is not going too well. Would you believe that nobody wants to hire an architect with twenty years' experience?

THERAPIST: I would think that expertise like that would be valuable.

JIM: Not in my case. Maybe they're afraid I'd be too set in my ways, or maybe they're afraid they'd have to pay too much even though I haven't made any demands. In fact, I can't even get past the receptionists. Lately I find myself almost paralyzed by fear every time I even think about arranging another interview. So instead, I go back to writing again.

JUDY: I keep telling him he should be more assertive. I mean, we're desperate here. We'll be into our retirement funds in another month.

JIM: And I keep telling her that if she's so smart, she should go out and find a job herself. She has *no idea* how it feels to get passed over in favor of some twenty-two-year-old fresh-out-of-school rookie. Knowing I'll get nagged when I walk in the door at home makes me want to stay away as long as possible.

JUDY: Yeah. Ask him where he goes. Tell her, Jim. The sports bar. He stops there every day, and comes home smelling like a brewery. No wonder he can't get up in the morning. No wonder we don't have enough money to pay the bills or for Heather to go out with her friends.

JIM: It's nowhere near what Judy's implying. I have a beer or two, sure, but mostly I just sit and watch sports on the big-screen TV, talk with my friends, and try to forget how it felt to get turned down again.

THERAPIST: A lot of guys handle their pain this way, Jim. But it can lead to trouble if you let it get out of control.

JIM: It won't. I'll keep trying. It's just hard to get up the courage again, and at least my friends there make me feel like I'm still worth something to someone.

THERAPIST: I understand, but next time we meet you might bring along a list of places where you've applied between now and then. If you haven't found a job by then, maybe we'll be able to come up with some creative alternatives together. *(turning to Judy)* Judy, Jim mentioned the possibility of you working. Is going to work an option for you?

JUDY: Not as far as I'm concerned. I quit college when our first child came, and I never went back. What kind of job could a person like me get in today's market?

THERAPIST: Jim, do you really want her to work?

JIM: Sure. That would be great. Having a job she liked might help her feel better about herself and take her mind off our situation. Of course, the money wouldn't hurt either.

JUDY: I'd rather finish my degree first. It would be a lot easier finding a good position if I had a degree.

JIM: Maybe, maybe not. My degree isn't worth diddly-squat. I should have studied something more practical or more technical.

THERAPIST: I have some good contacts in town in education and technology. Sometimes you can combine education or retraining with a work experience. I suggest that between this meeting and next you spend some time together establishing some goals—as a couple and personally. Have three columns—one for each of you, one for you together. Start from scratch. Let yourself dream again. Ask yourselves where you'd like to be five years from now in terms of your careers and personal lives. Then brainstorm what would have to happen in order to reach your goals individually and as a couple. We'll discuss these lists next time and use them as a basis for forming a plan. What do you think?

JIM: *(looking at the floor)* Sounds great, but I have to warn you that I feel pretty beat down and worthless right now.

JUDY: I think we should do it. Otherwise, we'll end up going in circles forever.[6]

Insight-Oriented (Psychodynamic) Therapy

Insight-oriented therapy seeks to identify the internal conflicts and psychological defenses that interfere with the depressed person's ability to love self and others. Experiences during childhood are often the focus of such therapy, since experiences or deprivations during the early years often establish repetitive patterns of behavior that endure throughout a person's life unless retraining occurs through conscious effort and new experiences. Achieving insight into the cause of one's anxiety, fears, anger, or self-condemnation can be emotionally freeing and help lift depression.

SESSION

THERAPIST: *(male psychologist)* Susan, you know in all the times we've talked you haven't said much about your childhood.

CLIENT: *(Silent. Sullen.)*

THERAPIST: Did you understand me?

CLIENT: *(Still silent. Finally speaks after another minute of silence.)* Did you need two weeks of vacation to come up with that question?

THERAPIST: Not necessarily. It had occurred to me earlier. You sound upset even though you knew I'd be gone.

CLIENT: I *am* upset—and rightly so. You left me on my own . . . just so you could have a good time!

THERAPIST: Do you recall feeling upset like this when you were a child?

CLIENT: Quite often, actually. I felt like this whenever I thought of my father and how he left us on our own just so he could have a good time and not be bothered with Mom and me anymore. Sometimes I tried to make him come back by hiding and refusing to come out even when Mom looked everywhere for me. I had a secret place.

THERAPIST: Tell me about that.

CLIENT: It was in a tree trunk on the bank of the stream behind our house. It was hollow on the downhill side, and the hole was big enough for me to climb inside.

THERAPIST: Weren't you afraid in there?

CLIENT: Not really. I liked it. It was the only place in the world I felt safe. It was dark and sometimes cold, but that's the way I felt most of the time—dark and cold. A squirrel shared that tree with me. He would sit on his branch chattering while I told him how I felt. Sometimes I would take him nuts, apples, or whatever.

THERAPIST: Can you tell *me* how you felt?

CLIENT: Mad. Hurt. Wounded. Empty, like there was a hole in my heart.

THERAPIST: Were you able to talk about this with anyone . . . for example, your mother?

CLIENT: Not really, she had enough problems. I never saw her smile after my father left. I wanted to help her, but what could I do? So we were sad together. Pretty soon she started drinking, and by the time I was a teenager I was stealing some of her whiskey every day, just to keep going. Swore I would never get married, but after she died I had nobody, and Jack swept me off my feet . . . and now he's gone, too.

THERAPIST: So it feels like everybody's abandoned you . . . and perhaps that nobody would care if you just ceased to exist?

CLIENT: Name one person who would miss me; one person who would even *know* that I was gone, much less *care* that I was gone.

THERAPIST: Well, I, for one, would care. And there are a lot of people here who would certainly miss you. But I'm wondering, was that what you were thinking the other night when you overdosed?

CLIENT: It wasn't intentional. I couldn't remember how many pills I had already taken. It was a mistake to add the whiskey, sure. But I just felt so lonely with no one to talk to. And you had been gone so long, and I . . .

THERAPIST: You wanted to punish me for going?

CLIENT: I didn't think of it that way. I guess I hoped that when they couldn't find me, it might make you come back. I remember crawling into that dark closet with my pills and my bottle and sitting there in the dark like I used to hide in my tree. But there was no squirrel and . . . well, I don't actually remember what happened after that.

THERAPIST: Nancy, from the half-way house, found you, and after a visit to the ER, you ended up here.

CLIENT: But even then you didn't come back.

THERAPIST: Dr. Bunaphali was available.

CLIENT: You're the only one who understands.

THERAPIST: I appreciate the sentiment, but overdosing is no way to make that point. We all want to understand and help you. In matters of the heart, there are no real experts, just fellow travelers willing to share your pain.

Group Psychotherapy

Group therapy can involve a variety of psychotherapeutic techniques described in this chapter. The goal of group therapy for people with depression is to help patients learn new skills and resources to better understand and address the causes of their depression. Group therapy is particularly helpful for people who share a common traumatic experience (such as bereavement, divorce, sexual or physical abuse, caregiver stress, etc.).

Members of the group learn to relate to, support, and validate each other. Many gain helpful insights into their own depression by listening to others describe theirs. Seeing others recover (or begin to recover) provides hope for those who still may feel stuck in their own personal pit of despair.

Usually, once a group has started, no new persons may join until all treatment sessions have been completed. Adding even one more person to this system of people changes all the relationships and in this context might significantly hinder progress by one or more participants.

Psychoanalysis

Psychoanalysis is a form of psychodynamic or insight-oriented therapy. Through a process called free association in which the patient talks and the analyst listens, the psychoanalyst attempts to help the patient uncover unconscious motivations and repressed memories so the person becomes more aware of how these affect his or her feelings and behavior. This process can sometimes take years.

Sigmund Freud was the father of psychoanalysis. In his view, depression (known in his day as "melancholia") was aggression turned inward in the form of anger at oneself. In his 1916 paper "Mourning and Melancholia," Freud distinguished between normal grief and melancholia. He wrote: "The distinguishing features of melancholia are a profoundly painful dejection, abrogation of interest in the outside world, loss of the capacity to love, inhibition of all activity, and a lowering of the self-regarding feelings to a degree that finds utterance in self-reproaches and self-revilings, and culminates in a delusional expectation of punishment."[7]

While it is certainly true that some degree of anger—both conscious and repressed—is often found in people who are depressed, it is unclear whether this anger is the cause or the result of the depression. Writing in 1982, Christian psychiatrist John White said, "The retroflexed-rage view of depression . . . remains a widely believed popular myth. Akiskal and McKinney comment, 'Even though this is the most widely quoted psychological conceptualization of depression, there is little systematic evidence to substantiate it.'" White adds that not only are Freud's theories difficult to prove, but they are also not very useful because therapists cannot make people better by applying his theories.[8] In fact, when depressed persons who are not already hostile are encouraged to direct their supposedly repressed rage outward, they do not get better; they get worse.

Conclusion

Based on what you've just read, it should be clear that there is a wide variety of counseling models and methods for treating depression. We have focused on the primary methods of talk therapy, which include cognitive, behavioral, cognitive-behavioral, interpersonal, marital, group, and insight-oriented psychotherapy, because these are the approaches that depressed people are most likely to encounter today.

Most of these approaches are more or less effective in treating depression. Some claim greater effectiveness than others, but the effectiveness of any particular approach may relate more to the combination of the therapist's skills and the client's personality than anything else.

The hypothetical counseling sessions provided a behind-closed-doors glimpse of what a depressed person might expect in a dialogue with therapists representing several of these perspectives. Our goal in providing these is to facilitate your process of selecting a counselor (and counseling method) that will be a good match for your personality and needs (see the guidelines on choosing a therapist at the end of this chapter).

Questions for Reflection

1. Review the various types of counseling described in this chapter. Which do you think might be most helpful for you or someone you care about who may be depressed?

2. Of the sessions in this chapter, which of them fits your situation more than the others did? (In other words, to whom did you feel closest?) List the reasons.

   Note: In a group situation, have two volunteers role-play the first session in which the counselor uses cognitive therapeutic approaches to help the businessman overcome his sense of failure when his work is less than perfect. After the role-play, let the actors describe what they learned by participating. Then have the group discuss how cognitive therapy might be helpful in counteracting negative thoughts that can fuel depression.

3. Why do you think that proponents of various models or methods of psychotherapy might have trouble seeing eye-to-eye?

4. How might the collaboration of various counselors benefit people with depression?

5. Do you think that secular therapists using the methods described in this chapter can benefit believers with depression? What deficits might exist in such a relationship? How might being treated by a secular therapist enable some believers to bring up deeply personal issues? How might secular psychotherapy be augmented for a believer by involving others in the treatment plan?

6. In cases in which anger is *contributing to* a person's depression, what is the best way to resolve it?

7. When anger is *resulting from* a person's depression, how can that situation be handled?

8. In your journal, write a letter to Susan (the suicidal woman in the last session) or to a person known to you who has issues similar to hers. Ask yourself: How can I connect this person with hope? Close your letter with a brief prayer for the person you've envisioned as you wrote.

Dreamweaving Checklist for Couples

Directions:

1. Each of you separately envision where you would like to be five years from now in terms of your careers and/or personal lives *without regard to current hindrances to these dreams.* Include as many relevant aspects as you wish.
2. Having done this separately, identify your shared long-term dreams or goals.
3. Brainstorm the steps necessary to achieve your goals. (For convenience we show five-year, three-year, one-year increments below—use any division that is most useful to you.)
4. Place all the relevant steps on a timeline (you may need a wide sheet or roll of paper for this).
5. Identify, as specifically as possible, how you will reach or achieve each step.
6. Decide together what your first steps will be and when you will begin.

	Her Goals	His Goals	Shared Goals
Long-term (5 years)			
Career/occupation			
Finances			
Education			
Relationships			
Spiritual life			
Other			
Medium-term (3 years)			
Career/occupation			
Finances			

Medium-term (3 years) *cont.*

Education

Relationships

Spiritual life

Other

Short-term (1 year)

Career/occupation

Finances

Education

Relationships

Spiritual life

Other

Time Line/Steps	One Year	Three Year	Five Year
How you plan to complete each step.			
Your first steps and when you'll begin.			

Choosing a Therapist

Suggestions and Guidelines

Overview: Once a decision has been reached that it would be best for a depressed person to obtain counseling, a caring and competent therapist must be found. We provide the following checklist as a starting point, knowing that no single checklist can provide options comprehensive enough to cover every situation. (Note that this material is repeated at the end of chapter 8, with a view toward choosing a Christian therapist.)

To begin with, we suggest that the selection of a counselor not be made individually (unless there is no other choice). The support and wisdom of family, friends, and/or trusted advisors combined with the advice of one's attending physician can identify a variety of issues for consideration that may not occur to a single individual, especially a depressed person seeking help.

Your physician may be able to provide a list of possible therapists. Also, the names of potential therapists sometimes can be generated by polling friends who are known to have had positive experiences with counselors in your area. However, keep in mind that any referral only represents the referring person's opinion and/or experience, and the goal in the selection process is to find the right counselor for the depressed person.

The following questions may help identify the right counselor in a given case:

1. What models or methods seem to match the needs in this case (see "Counseling Models and Methods" at the beginning of this chapter)?

2. What type of training, experience, and/or certification/licensing is preferred (check one)? (You may wish to review chapter 6.)
   - ☐ counselor/therapist (unlicensed/uncertified)
   - ☐ licensed/certified social worker
   - ☐ licensed/certified psychologist
   - ☐ licensed/certified psychiatrist

3. Will the counselor be expected to prescribe and monitor medications if needed? If so, the person ordinarily must be a physician or a licensed/certified mental health professional working under the supervision of a physician (M.D. or D.O., including psychiatrists).

4. How will the expenses be paid? If via medical insurance, the list of approved providers may considerably limit options available. By comparing this list with lists of counselors and/or physicians via the various web sites listed in chapters 6 and 7, you may be able to find one or more matches.

5. Does the gender of the counselor make a difference to the person in question?

The remaining questions are best answered via conversation with potential counselors, most of whom will either meet you in person at no charge or agree to an interview by phone.

1. Are the client's and counselor's personalities compatible?

2. Is the counselor compassionate, understanding, and willing to listen, or condescending, arrogant, judgmental, or overconfident?

3. Does the counselor have any special clinical experience that might relate to this case beyond the minimum required for his or her certification?

4. Is the counselor a team player, or does he or she give the impression that his or her help can take care of all problems related to this case?

5. What is the counselor's primary counseling model and method?

6. What are the counselor's views regarding the value of antidepressants?

7. Does the counselor have (or at least respect) a whole-person view of the causes and cures for depression?

8. What are the counselor's charges? How and when will he or she expect to be paid?

9. How many sessions are usually required, and how long do individual sessions last?

10. Where will the counseling be conducted?

11. What office hours does the counselor normally keep?

12. Will anyone else be present in the office (for example, a receptionist)?

13. What kind of records will be kept (for example, sessions taped, handwritten notes, etc.)?

14. Who will have access to these records?

15. What arrangements does the therapist have for emergency needs after hours?

CHAPTER 8

Models and Methods
of Christian Counseling

W e begin this chapter with the true story of one person's experience with several Christian counselors who used a wide
variety of methods, not all of which were helpful. While this
case is unusual in some ways, it illustrates the diversity that exists in
Christian counseling today.

Happy Housewife

Prior to April 1993, thirty-six-year-old LezLee Guy's life was all that any
Christian housewife could ask. With a husband, Richard, who loved her,
and two children, Rich, sixteen, and Nicholle, fourteen, LezLee was
expecting them all to live happily ever after. Then, like a hellish nightmare, her husband died from a pulmonary embolism. Two months later,
while LezLee and the children were traveling by car to visit the ceme-
tery on Father's Day, an eighty-one-year-old woman lost control of her
car and careened into the Guys' car. Nicholle was killed instantly.

Absolutely devastated and in shock, LezLee reached out for help
from a counselor associated with her church. This therapist was usually
nondirective,[1] expecting LezLee to carry the conversation week after
week even though she had little energy to do so. Once, however, he
asked her to pretend that Richard was sitting there with them, which
was impossible for LezLee at that time due to her deteriorating condition—clinical depression, posttraumatic stress disorder, panic attacks,
and an eating disorder as a result of which she would ultimately lose
eighty-five pounds. She was taking at least a dozen prescription pills a
day in addition to the sleeping pills she mixed with alcohol. Finally, this

155

therapist convinced her to admit herself to the psychiatric ward of a local hospital, the first of half a dozen hospitals to which she would be admitted over time, twice for the eating disorder and the others due to suicide attempts.

LezLee's second Christian counselor saved her life by calling for help during her last suicide attempt, just before Christmas 1996. "He was awesome as a counselor," LezLee said. "I knew he cared. He would cry with me from time to time. Once after leaving his office, I had a panic attack right outside in the hallway. He came out there and sat down with me—he always met me wherever I was at—until I was able to leave. He used Scripture sometimes, but he never threw it at me. Sometimes he offered advice I didn't like but I needed to hear.[2] He was totally dependable, and I always felt secure with him."

LezLee's third Christian counselor saw her briefly after she moved to Colorado in 1997. But this college professor/counselor felt that another counselor would be better for LezLee, so he referred her to a woman who specialized in "prayer therapy."

This fourth Christian counselor made it clear that prayer was all she did. "She believed that the only way people can be healed is through the Holy Spirit," LezLee said. "So we prayed through the whole session, every time. I should say that *she* prayed. I couldn't pray then, so the whole thing left me feeling extremely uncomfortable."

LezLee's fifth Christian counselor had lost his wife to cancer several years prior to LezLee's first meeting him. "He is so real," LezLee said. "He understands. He tries to help his clients find purpose and meaning in their experiences."[4]

Each of the counselors who saw LezLee used the method of counseling with which he or she was most familiar. Some used methods like those described in chapter 7. Some used more spiritually oriented methods, like those described in this chapter. Some helped; some didn't—the latter probably because the method did not match very well LezLee's condition and needs.[5]

Christian Counseling Models and Methods

General Christian Combines insights from secular counseling with relevant biblical principles to help clients toward wholeness.[3] May use nondirective, directive, or interactive approaches.

Nouthetic Exhorts client to pattern thoughts and actions according to the counselor's understanding of a biblical model. Usually directive.

R.E.S.T. Rational-emotive spiritual therapy focuses on helping individuals break self-destructive habits and gain control of negative controlling emotions. Usually interactive.

Theophostic Helps emotionally wounded people find emotional and spiritual freedom through a personal encounter with the Spirit of Jesus Christ. May use nondirective, directive, or interactive approaches.

Some Christian counseling models incorporate the more helpful elements of models described in chapter 7. For example, a Christian form of cognitive therapy that employs Scripture to challenge maladaptive thinking is described in self-help books such as *Telling Yourself the Truth* and *Slaying the Giant*.[6] Christian therapists will often use this approach to treat those with depression or anxiety. The client learns how to counter negative thoughts about the self with positive biblical concepts such as, "I am a child of God because God the Father chose me long ago." Or, "I have the Holy Spirit at work in my heart, making me pleasing to God." Similarly, some Christian therapists use behavioral therapy to reinforce behaviors that are Christlike and affirming of self and others. Other Christian counseling models claim to totally reject any input from secular psychology, sticking instead to what they call "biblical counseling." Whatever their approach may be, counselors who are most effective are those who have the ability to offer depressed people hope.

General Christian Counseling

Psychologist Gary Collins, Ph.D., was a pioneer in this field. The introduction to one of his many books says, "In approaching the aspects of life that are discussed in the following pages I have been guided by three considerations: my personal observations as a clinical psychologist, a review of the contemporary psychological literature, and a consideration of what the Bible says about man and his emotions.[7]

Collins's work helped establish the contemporary model of Christian counseling.[8] Later on, the Christian counseling movement began to pick up speed and the American Association of Christian Counselors was formed, consisting of certified Christian counselors.[9] There is also a National Christian Counselors Association, consisting of professional counselors who receive special training in Christian counseling and become certified by this national organization.[10] Yet another group is the American Association of Christian Therapists, which provides training and certification for professional Christian counselors.[11] Each of these groups trains Christian counselors from a slightly different perspective.

Nouthetic Counseling (NC)

NC is a form of biblical counseling developed by Jay Adams, Ph.D., in the 1970s. This form of Christian counseling, which does not require a counseling degree, arose from Adams's best-selling *Competent to Counsel* and is used by the National Association of Nouthetic Counselors (NANC), the Christian Counseling and Educational Foundation, and the Biblical Counseling Foundation. Taken from the NANC web site, NC is described by Dr. Adams as follows: "The three ideas found in the [Greek] word *nouthesia* are Confrontation, Concern, and Change. To put it simply, nouthetic counseling consists of lovingly confronting people out of deep concern in order to help them make those changes that God requires. By confrontation we mean that one Christian personally gives counsel to another from the Scriptures. He does not confront him with his own ideas or the ideas of others. He claims to limit his counsel strictly to that which may be found in the Bible."[12]

Adams and others have spoken strongly against Christian counseling that combines secular psychotherapeutic techniques with biblical principles.[13] Although nouthetic counseling claims to be strictly biblical, it does have its critics—primarily because how one interprets and uses the Bible in counseling depends greatly upon one's *theological perspective.*[14]

NC proponents interpret the Bible from the perspective of covenant theology, which applies many Old Testament (the word *testament* means "covenant") passages to Christians today as if the New Testament church is the new people of God (as the people of Israel were in the Old Testament). However, this approach can be quite selective, as some of the Old Testament law is ignored while other parts are promoted as counseling gems. Certain portions of the Old Testament, Proverbs for example, contain concepts or teachings that are obviously general principles for guidance in faith (most likely aimed at teaching these principles to the young). To pick and choose and then to apply a particular wisdom nugget directly to individual twenty-first century Christians is not consistent with good exegesis (biblical interpretation), which requires that certain questions be answered before such applications are made. These questions include: "To/for whom was this written?" "What would it have meant to them?" and "Are there any timeless directives, principles, or lessons to be derived from this passage?" In the context of the answers to the first questions, inquiries such as: "What does the passage mean to the church today?" or "What does it say to individual twenty-first century believers?" and other similar issues may be pursued.

"Nouthetic counselors frequently hand out individual portions of the book of Proverbs," Adams writes.

One reason why they have found Proverbs so useful in counseling is that essentially it is a book of good counsel given to covenant youth. Proverbs was written primarily to promote divine wisdom among God's covenant people. It anticipates the pitfalls and problems of life and directs the reader to make biblical responses to them. Proverbs capsulizes segments of life as God expects his children to live it in a sinful world. . . .

In nouthetic counseling the book of Proverbs plays a very significant part because these proverbs give instruction. The system of counseling advocated in Proverbs is plainly nouthetic. Proverbs assumes the need for divine wisdom imparted by verbal means: by instruction, by reproof, by rebuke, by correction, and by applying God's commandments in order to change behavior for one's benefit.[15]

In terms of NC's understanding of depression, Adams says,

Thus, nouthetic counselors adhere closely to the principle enunciated in Proverbs 28:13: He who conceals his transgressions will not prosper, but he who confesses and forsakes them will receive mercy (Berkeley) and confidently assure their clients that in this way they may find mercy from God. This methodology is biblical methodology; it is therefore certain and sure. It is fitting to and grows out of the fundamental nouthetic principle that man's problems stem from sin. Depressed persons whose symptoms fail to show any sign of a biochemical root should be counseled on the assumption that they are depressed by guilt.[16]

The key phrases, in terms of the scope of our book, are "the system of counseling advocated in Proverbs" and "depressed persons whose symptoms fail to show any sign of a biochemical root should be counseled on the assumption that they are depressed by guilt." Regarding the former, our perspective is that *no* system of counseling is advocated in Proverbs. Proverbs is a collection of wise sayings, the application of which helps a person grow in wisdom while avoiding thoughts and actions that are foolish. Proverbs is in no way a handbook for the diagnosis and treatment of clinical depression. Further, we believe that while some nonbiochemical depressions are a result of guilt, not all of them fit this model. To force a person whose depression springs from another source through this knothole is not in his or her best interest.

In any case, if you choose to see a nouthetic biblical counselor for depression, you can expect to be confronted about your sins and encouraged to repent in order to find healing through God's mercy and release from the guilt that is making you depressed. You may receive printed

We do not believe that the Proverbs were intended by God to serve as a handbook for counseling clinically depressed persons.

Bible verses to memorize and put into practice. Assuming that the verses provided are relevant to your needs, this practice is fine, except when it is accompanied by unwarranted claims about its efficacy and unwarranted promises this discipline is all you need in order to cure your depression.

There are many varieties of biblical interpretation—such as reformed, dispensational, and so forth—all of which approach the Scripture with theological presuppositions and none of which can possibly have it all right all the time. So calling oneself a "biblical counselor" means very little unless one is also forthright about the particular systematic theology that provides the glasses through which the counselor in question normally views particular portions of Scripture.

To be clear, we believe that God's Word is truth, as Jesus said. We also believe that God's "power has given us everything we need for life and godliness through our knowledge of him who called us by his own glory and goodness" (2 Peter 1:3).[17] We do not believe, however, that the Proverbs were intended by God to serve as a handbook for counseling (specifically, in our context, for counseling clinically depressed persons). The Bible, it seems clear to us, is our handbook for faith and godliness. While the Bible's truth intersects questions related to clinical depression at various points, other factors must be considered as well if we embrace a truly holistic model of human nature.

The Bible is truth, yet it nowhere claims to describe everything that is true. Scientific method has discovered many true things that are neither within the purview of nor antithetic to the truth found in the Scriptures. In the context of depression, this includes methods for assessing the degree of a person's depression, whether or not there may be a biochemical root in a particular case, and which methods really help certain disorders. Our belief is that as long as the treatment itself does not contradict Scripture, the use of modern science to treat depression is certainly as acceptable an appropriation of truth as handing out portions of Proverbs to one's counselees.

Rational-Emotive Spiritual Therapy (R.E.S.T.)

According to this group's web site, this form of spiritual counseling, often provided by lay counselors who view themselves as guides, "utilizes a combination of biblical principles of healing and humanistic counseling in conjunction with the accumulated knowledge and understandings of the intricate relationship between the mind, body, and emotions (feelings, thoughts, and behaviors)."[18] R.E.S.T. focuses especially on helping individuals break self-destructive habits and gain control of negative controlling emotions. Adherents believe that learned behavior can be unlearned, including addictions to substances and related antisocial behavior.

This form of spiritual counseling borrows from numerous secular models and methods, including rational-emotive therapy, a technique developed by Albert Ellis, a well-known atheist who viewed religion as emotionally destabilizing. In R.E.S.T., a group of Christian therapists have taken his theories (and others) and combined them with biblical principles.

We're not sure we should recommend this therapy for persons with more than mild depression, because although R.E.S.T. claims to be holistic, its primary focus seems to be faith healing of spiritual illness. Its counselors are admittedly ignorant about psychological theories and methodologies, according to the web site. Thus, they likely would not recognize major depression or refer clients with major depression for appropriate treatment. Indeed, their efforts could intensify the struggles of someone who is clinically depressed from biological causes.

We do believe the Holy Spirit can bring supernatural healing to a depressed person's soul—surely a form of supernatural healing. However, we also believe that this type of healing for clinically depressed persons most often occurs in the context of a multifaceted treatment effort addressing his or her biological, psychological, sociological, and spiritual deficits.

> *Supernatural healing of clinically depressed persons most often occurs in the context of a multifaceted treatment effort addressing his or her biological, psychological, sociological, and spiritual deficits.*

Theophostic Ministry (TM)

Described on their web site as a Christian counseling ministry, theophostic (Greek: *theo* = God; *phostic* = light) strives to "help emotionally wounded people find freedom through a personal encounter with the Spirit of Christ."[19] The idea is that people who are experiencing emotional distress often have been wounded by events or experiences in their past (for example, a person who was raped or abused as a child). That negative experience and the feelings associated with it are suppressed during childhood but find expression when the person experiences similar events in adult life (for example, when attempting to be intimate with a spouse). The theophostic minister helps the person identify the

Theophostic ministers help clients resolve long-standing distress through an encounter with the Spirit of Christ.

traumatic event or experience and then leads the person through a process whereby Jesus Christ brings healing to that experience or memory. TM claims that once such healing has occurred, people are totally freed of the emotional distress brought on by the original event and all future similar events that typically evoke negative responses.

A Christian psychiatrist described how he used theophostic methods with a long-time patient, a social worker. The patient and his wife had nearly lost their first child to a rare disease, which required multiple surgeries, radiation, chemotherapy, and a bone marrow transplant after relapse. The couple had watched the child almost die so many times that they were both worn out and depressed. Just at the time when the diagnosis of the child's illness was made, the father had been dealing with some memories of sexual abuse by two priests that had started when he was a student at a Catholic boarding school. With both crises occurring simultaneously, this man felt hit with a double whammy, as a result of which he went to God with the rage and confusion of it all.

"Where there was bitterness and rage there is now forgiveness," the psychiatrist said. "Where there was confusion there is now some clearing of the clouds. And the deep sadness has gradually given way to joy again.

"To me," he added, "secular therapies talk around or about bitterness and rage, gradually chipping away at it. But in this man's case, the process was much more direct. We went to a memory many years after the abuse when my patient had been chopping wood in the back yard. He had been imagining that the priests' heads were on the blocks as they were split.

"Are you tired of the bitterness?" I asked. "Would you like Jesus to help you with this burden?"

"Yes," he said, "I am finally ready."

"At that moment, the Lord Jesus showed himself to my client in the memory in question. And when he handed Jesus the axe, it was changed into a cross in the Master's hands. Jesus helped my client forgive the priests, leaving their disposition up to God. Then the Lord interposed the cross between the man and the priests, with the result that thoughts of them never come up anymore. Jesus gave my client a hug and let him know he would never leave or forsake him. The patient experienced real relief of the bitterness, anger, confusion, loneliness, and sadness that had lingered for so long. My job as intercessor was simply to bring my client to Jesus; after that I was mostly silent in this most remarkable session.

"I have learned to quiet myself," the psychiatrist concluded, "not to spout human wisdom or Bible verses, when the Living Word is himself in the room. Not everyone receives answers quite this way; some hear only a still, small voice . . . which is just as true and healing."

TM is a rapidly growing form of ministry in the United States. Dr. Ed Smith founded this ministry in the late 1990s. He offers seminars and a video training program to people who wish to become theophostic ministers. He claims that this ministry can be done by anyone who completes his video course (including those without counseling experience or certification).

Although Smith claims that TM is not counseling, I (HK) have taken the training program and feel that this is a good form of Christian counseling for people with specific life traumas in their past that are affecting their present functioning. When these are contributing to mild depression, their relief should bring improvement. In more severe cases, however, we feel this type of ministry should be administered or supervised by a mental health professional familiar with the symptoms and treatment of clinical depression.

Creative Imagery, Visualization, and Related Methods

We believe that any type of psychotherapy involving creative imagery, visualization, and related methods should be conducted by a trained professional who is also a mature Christian, since the state of the patient in such an exercise may leave him or her open to suggestions by the therapist that might alter the memories in question. Some would consign the use of these methods to the realm of the occult in which sorcerers conjure up a false Jesus, who acts as spirit guide leading the participant away from, not toward, truth. These critics insist that the love and forgiveness of God—who indwells, controls, and empowers every true believer—should be totally adequate as our model and means to love and forgive others as God, for Christ's sake, has forgiven us. They see journeying back into the memory for any purpose as unnecessary or worse since in Christ all things have been made new and all that should matter now is one's relationship with him.

While we understand these objections and would certainly agree that walking through any experience with a "Jesus" created by one's own imagination would be worse than futility, we are not convinced that the use of creative imagery and related therapies are necessarily destructive to one's spirit. This opinion is based, in part, on the testimonies of so many who have experienced healing and release through these methods, followed by a subsequent growth in Christian character, love for the Lord, and faithful involvement in his ongoing work of redemption in the world. If the experience were a counterfeit inspired by the Deceiver, we doubt that he would be very satisfied with this result.

Although the Bible itself does not contain anything specific about this method, it does contain a great deal of creative imagery that was guided or inspired by God. For example, David wrote, "The LORD is my shepherd, I shall not be in want" (Ps. 23:1). Of course the Lord is not a shepherd, per se. This is a poet's creative attempt to bring people of faith toward a deeper understanding of God and the intensely personal relationship he wishes to have with his "sheep."

When Elijah tried to discern God's voice, he did not hear it in the earthquake or in the fire but as a "gentle whisper" addressing him in the quietness of his mind or spirit (1 Kings 19:11–13). Did God appear to Moses in the form of a burning bush that was not consumed because he wanted his people forever to imagine him this way, or was he trying to say, by analogy, something profound about his character? Did Jesus literally mean, "I am the door" (John 10:9 NASB), or "I am the vine" (John 15:1–8), or was he appealing to the creative image of God instilled in all humans and enlightened by his Spirit to understand his deeper meanings?

One of the unaddressed problems for the critics of creative imaging in all its varieties is the fact that God dwells in the eternal present, so their emphasis on the tenses of the person's journey may be irrelevant to God. As the Scripture says, "Jesus Christ is the same yesterday and today and forever" (Heb. 13:8). This was the meaning of God's statement, when Moses asked his name and God said, "I AM WHO I AM. This is what you are to say to the Israelites: 'I AM has sent me to you'" (Ex. 3:14).[20] In other words, God is the source of all being, or as he put it later, "I am the Alpha and the Omega [first and last letters of the Greek alphabet] . . . who is, and who was, and who is to come, the Almighty" (Rev. 1:8; see also Rev. 21:6; 22:13).

In light of God's own assertions about his relationship to what we call time, we believe it possible that he is able to move with a person from the *now* of their experience back in time to their prior experiences, because to him it is all the same, for he was there then as he is here now. Some believers even assert that God can move backward and forward in time at will, which, if true, may have some relevance for counseling using this method. For example, one might ask clients to project themselves to the end of their lives, considering what they would want the Lord to say to them in the afterlife or perhaps how they would like to be remembered. Both questions have implications for how they should lead their lives from now onward.

The assertion that the past is irrelevant to God (or to any believer) is not consistent with how Jesus handled related questions when they arose. For example, when he spoke with the woman at the well, who said she had no husband, Jesus revealed in a lovingly confrontational way that he knew that she had had five husbands and that she was not married to the one with whom she was living at the moment. He was exhorting her to leave her life of sin and move ahead by faith in him as the Messiah (see John 4:7–26). Had the woman's past been irrelevant, Jesus certainly would not have mentioned it. He could just as easily have said, as he said to some others, "Come. Follow me."

In another case, when Jesus met Peter soon after the resurrection, the Lord could have put his arm around the disciple who had recently denied him three times and said something like, "Peter, my friend, the past doesn't matter. Let's just forget the fact that you denied me three times and get on with the task of feeding my sheep." Instead the Lord mirrored Peter's triple denial with a question asked three times in slightly different form: "Do you love me?" By handling the situation this way, Jesus took the guilty Peter back to the event and let him know he was forgiven. Jesus also used creative imagery to give him the commission that would occupy the rest of his life: "Feed my lambs. . . . Take care of my sheep. . . . Feed my sheep" (John 21:15–19).

Yes, we are all to press on toward the mark of the higher calling in Christ, forgetting what has gone before, reaching for what lies ahead (see Phil. 3:12–14). Yet the apostle Paul, who penned these words, occasionally referred in his writings to his past persecution of the church and even to his participation in murdering believers. We know that he was present at the death of the church's first martyr, Stephen. Paul refers to himself as the "worst of sinners" (speaking of sins that had occurred in the past) in order to show, by contrast, the transforming and redemptive power of the grace of God. The past truly is important, especially when it is a mirror to show us how God is working in our lives today.

When Paul spoke in Philippians 3:1–14 of forgetting what has gone before, he wasn't just speaking of his past sins. He was very specifically speaking of his past "righteous" achievements under the Law, including his position as a Pharisee, which, compared to the value of knowing

Christ, the apostle counted as "dung." If the past should have no relevance for believers, then Paul probably would not have referred to either his past sins or, indeed, to his past perceived righteousness.

To deny that we are all products of our past is to ignore the importance of our individuality. We are not, after all, to be cookie-cutter Christians—clones of some other human's image of normalcy—but we are to be remade, through God's Spirit, into the likeness of Christ. In God's view it is our differences, including the depths from which we have been rescued and the variety of gifts bestowed by his Spirit, that contribute to the multifaceted personality of the body of Christ representing him today in this world.[21]

For some people forgetting what has gone before is a process, not an event, through which they release others and, more importantly, *release themselves* from the prison of bitterness or guilt that is preventing them from being all they can be in Christ. Going backward in time—if that is really what is occurring here—with Christ as one's guide is a means to an end (forgiveness), not a method for blaming our present problems on someone in our past.

We believe the use of creative imagery, visualization, role-playing, and related methods to achieve this end are not necessarily contrary to God's will or his Word, in which he often uses creative images to try to communicate who he is. Jesus demonstrated in person what God is like, and in John 16:7–23 as he prepared to leave his disciples so another "Counselor" (some versions read "Comforter"—he was referring to the Holy Spirit) could come, he said: "I tell you the truth, you will weep and mourn while the world rejoices. You will grieve, but your grief will turn to joy. . . . I will see you again and you will rejoice, and no one will take away your joy" (vv. 20, 22).

Questions for Reflection

1. LezLee (introductory case) was seen by a variety of counselors, some of whom were helpful, some not. If you were her, what characteristics would you need in a counselor in order to connect enough to resolve some of the pain?

2. Some counselors claim to use the Bible as a handbook for counseling depressed persons. What are the advantages or disadvantages of this counseling model—to the counselor; to the client?

3. The proponents of R.E.S.T. believe that God can bring spiritual healing through their methods. If you find this approach attractive, explain why. If you think it has significant deficiencies, what would they be?

4. Some Christian therapists use creative visualization and similar methods in order to facilitate inner healing/healing of memories. List values and/or dangers of this method.

5. What word comes to mind when you think of trying to find the "right" counselor?

6. Record in your journal at least one way that your struggle with depression could result in something good. Pray (even write the prayer down if you wish) that this will indeed take place.

Choosing a Christian Therapist

Suggestions and Guidelines

For believers, the search for the *right* counselor may be more or less complicated by the question of whether or not to seek Christian counseling, and if so, what type of Christian counseling would be preferred. The following guidelines (a revised version of the guidelines at the end of chapter 7) should help patients, their families, friends, clergy, and other advisors reach an informed and wise decision.

The patient's physician may be able to provide a list of trusted therapists. If the physician is a believer, these therapists may be Christians, supportive of the role of faith in one's overall health, and willing to be part of a cooperative treatment team.

Names of effective Christian counselors may come via friends or others in the area who have had good experiences with Christian counseling. Names of certified Christian counselors also may be found on the web site of the Christian Counseling Center Referral Network.[22] Again, keep in mind that any referral only represents the referring person's opinion and/or experience, and the goal in the selection process is to find the right counselor for *the depressed person*.

The following questions may help identify the right counselor in this case:

1. What type of treatment is being sought: medical, psychological, sociological, spiritual, or a combination?
2. What models or methods seem to match the needs in this case (see "Christian Counseling and Modeling Methods" earlier in this chapter)?
3. Does the client feel more comfortable with a nondirective, directive, or interactive approach from the counselor?
4. What type of training, experience, and/or certification/licensing is preferred? (Circle your preference.)
   - [ ] General Christian counselor (unlicensed/uncertified)—may include clergy or church staff counselor
   - [ ] General Christian counselor (certified or licensed)—combining secular and spiritual treatment methods
   - [ ] Pastoral counselor (certified/licensed)—clergy with specific training in counseling
   - [ ] Nouthetic counselor—focused primarily on application of biblical truth to life; may have training in this method, but usually no state-recognized certification/licensing
   - [ ] R.E.S.T. counselor—unlicensed, but some training in this method
   - [ ] Theophostic counselor—may have training in this method, but often no state-recognized certification/licensing
5. Will the counselor be expected to prescribe and monitor medications if needed? If so, the person ordinarily must be a physician or a licensed/certified mental health professional working under the supervision of a physician (M.D. or D.O., including psychiatrists).
6. How will the expenses be paid? If via medical insurance, the list of approved providers may considerably limit options available. By comparing this list with lists of

counselors and/or physicians via the various web sites listed in chapters 6 and 7, you may be able to find one or more matches.

7. Does the gender of the counselor make a difference to the person in question?

The remaining questions are best answered via conversation with potential counselors, most of whom will either meet with you in person at no charge or agree to an interview by phone.

1. Are the client's and counselor's personalities compatible?
2. Is the counselor compassionate, understanding, and willing to listen, or condescending, arrogant, judgmental, or overconfident?
3. Does the counselor have any special clinical experience that might relate to this case, beyond the minimum required for his or her certification?
4. Is the counselor a team player, or does he or she give the impression that his or her help can take care of all problems related to this case?

5. What is the counselor's primary counseling model and method?
6. What are the counselor's views regarding the value of antidepressants?
7. Does the counselor have (or at least respect) a whole-person (biopsychosociospiritual) view of depression's causes and cures?
8. What are the counselor's charges? How and when will he or she expect to be paid?
9. How many sessions are usually required, and how long do individual sessions last?
10. Where will the counseling be conducted?
11. What office hours does the counselor normally keep?
12. Will anyone else be present in the office (for example, a receptionist)?
13. What kind of records will be kept (for example, sessions taped, handwritten notes, etc.)?
14. Who will have access to the records kept?
15. What arrangements does the therapist have for emergency needs after hours?

CHAPTER 9

Antidepressant Medications
What They Are and How They Work

Forrest Jones facilitates a depression support group sponsored by Lookout Mountain Community Church in Golden, Colorado. Over the past several years he has led or participated in more than ten such groups. Without exception during the time the group meets—usually weekly for three or four months—fellow pilgrims who started out as strangers become close friends, in part due to Forrest's sensitive leadership. The changes in and between the participants are remarkable in themselves, but perhaps even more remarkable is the fact that as recently as 1999, the facilitator was so depressed he couldn't even get out of bed. Here is his story in his own words:

"In retrospect," Forrest said, "I can see that I've had some symptoms of depression most of my life. But about three years ago three unrelated events happened in succession, and this triggered my first major depression—my mother died, I turned fifty, and I quit a job I loved because I didn't see eye-to-eye with my supervisor.

"Over the next year, I gradually slid into the muck of despair. For the first six months I was barely functional. Then it just seemed that my energy left. I could hardly get out of bed. I felt so alone, worthless, mired in misery and emotional pain. I even prayed to die.

171

"I sensed that my marriage was suffering, and that just added to my feelings of worthlessness. Finally my wife, Connie, confronted me, saying, 'Something has to change. You can't go on like this. You have to get help.'

"Asking for help was the hardest thing I've ever done, partly due to my pride," Forrest continued. "After all, I've been a Christian forty years. Shouldn't I be able to help myself?

"Providentially, only two days after I decided to ask for help, a depression support group was started in a local church. I'll never forget that first meeting because when I walked in, my primary feeling was that I would rather be *anywhere* other than there. I didn't want to have to describe my struggles, but it was clear from the outset that the room was occupied by a group of special people, each with his or her own story, most of them a lot like my own. *So, maybe I'm not so strange,* I thought. From that night on, hope took root in my heart . . . hope that I might someday experience joy again.

"The other thing that happened that night was equally difficult for me. The topic of antidepressant medication came up again and again. *I'd rather be dead than have to take drugs for this,* was my thought. 'But the right medication will help you think more clearly,' I heard, 'and this will speed your healing.' 'You'd have to stand on me and shove the pills down my throat,' I said. However, the Lord convicted me that if I really wanted to recover, I had to stop insisting that it be on my own terms.

"My physician started me on an antidepressant, which I took for five or six weeks before telling him that it was helping a little, but my life was still mostly gray. He doubled the dosage, and within days the difference was like night and day. Life was beautiful again, in living color. I was happy to be alive.

"It took a long time and the help of a psychiatrist to settle on the right combination of drugs that would most help me. During this long journey, several things have become clear to me: (1) The Lord can use my struggle to help others. (2) Most people who are afflicted with depression are compassionately sensitized to the suffering of others. (3) With today's advanced medications, there is no reason that *anyone* should slog sadly along in silence as I did for a year, because there is healing to be had."

How Antidepressants Work

Because depression can have strong biological roots, medication or other biological therapies may be necessary and can be lifesaving. Just like certain types of diabetes require insulin and high blood pressure requires antihypertensive medications, depression may require drugs to help reset the imbalance of brain chemicals that occurs in this disease. The most common and widely used biological treatments for depression are antidepressant drugs. There are currently about twenty such medications available, with new ones being released on a regular basis.

Antidepressants are not uppers or stimulants. They do not bend the mind, but they help to straighten it. Antidepressants lift depression's symptoms by correcting or compensating for a malfunction in the patient's body that has impaired his or her ability to function normally. For people who have been suffering with depression for a long time, these treatments can be remarkably helpful, sometimes bringing them back to life in a matter of weeks.

Antidepressants work by increasing the level of neurotransmitters in certain parts of the brain necessary to maintain positive mood and attitudes. Neurotransmitters are chemical messengers in brain tissue that allow brain cells (neurons) to communicate with one another. If these chemicals (serotonin, norepinephrine, dopamine, and others) become depleted in key brain areas, a person begins to feel tired, sad, and unhappy. Antidepressants increase levels of neurotransmitters in the brain by either preventing their breakdown or by making brain cells more sensitive to their actions.

Some people inherit lower levels of neurotransmitters necessary to maintain mood or their brain cells are less sensitive to the actions of these chemicals. Some with long-term psychological conflict due to negative experiences during infancy or childhood can also experience a drop in the levels of key neurotransmitters, resulting in depression. Severe stress in adulthood may likewise deplete or reduce brain neurotransmitters. Some people might say after a period of prolonged stress that they "feel burned out," which is a fairly good description of what happens as his or her level of neurotransmitters decreases, resulting in depression or feelings of exhaustion. This is also why some doctors explain depression as a "chemical imbalance." Antidepressants help to restore the equilibrium of neurotransmitters in the brain, facilitating normal mood function.

Antidepressants help to restore the equilibrium of neurotransmitters in the brain, facilitating normal mood function.

Types of Antidepressants

There are several different classes of antidepressants, depending on which neurotransmitter the medication affects most: norepinephrine, serotonin, dopamine, or small proteins out of which these chemicals are made (called neurotransmitter precursors). Medications affecting

Monoamine Oxidase Inhibitors (MAOIs)

Norepinephrine and serotonin are normally destroyed by the enzyme monoamine oxidase (MAO). MAO inhibitors block this enzyme, inhibiting the destruction of norepinephrine and serotonin, allowing the neurotransmitters to remain active longer.

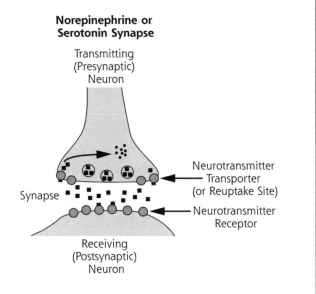

Norepinephrine or Serotonin Synapse

Transmitting (Presynaptic) Neuron

Neurotransmitter Transporter (or Reuptake Site)

Neurotransmitter Receptor

Synapse

Receiving (Postsynaptic) Neuron

Diagrams © Keith A. Trujillo, Ph.D. Used with permission. Taken from: *www.csusm.edu/psychology/DandB/AD.html.*

norepinephrine include the tricyclic compounds desipramine, nortriptyline, and maprotiline (Ludiomil). Those affecting serotonin are called SSRIs and include fluoxetine, paroxetine, sertraline, fluvoxamine (Luvox), and citalopram. Antidepressants that affect both norepinephrine and serotonin include amitriptyline, doxepine, imipramine, and venlafaxine. The only antidepressant that primarily affects dopamine is bupropion. Antidepressants that have uncertain mechanisms of action on brain cell receptors include mirtazapine and nefazadone. Those with mixed action (affecting a variety of different brain chemicals) include clomipramine (Anafranil), amoxapine (Asendin), and trazodone.

Monoamine oxidase inhibitors (MAOIs) inactivate enzymes in the brain that break down the neurotransmitter precursors such as tyramine. MAOIs include phenelzine (Nardil) and tranylcypromine (Parnate). The first MAOI, iproniazid, was removed from the market because of toxic effects on the liver (the MAOIs prescribed today do not have that effect). Both phenelzine and tranylcypromine, however, may interact with certain foods and drugs to increase blood pressure to dangerous levels. For example, if a person taking an MAOI eats a diet rich

Transmitting (Presynaptic Neuron) Tricyclic Antidepressants

Norepinephrine and serotonin are normally removed from the synapse by reuptake sites. Tricyclic antidepressants block norepinephrine and serotonin reuptake sites, allowing these neurotransmitters to remain active in the synapse longer.

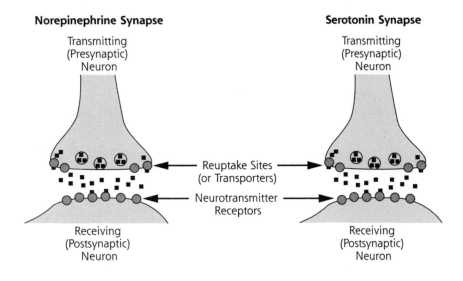

Serotonin Reuptake Inhibitors (SSRIs)

Serotonin is normally removed from the synapse by reuptake sites on the presynaptic neuron. SSRIs block the serotonin reuptake sites, allowing serotonin to remain active in the synapse longer.

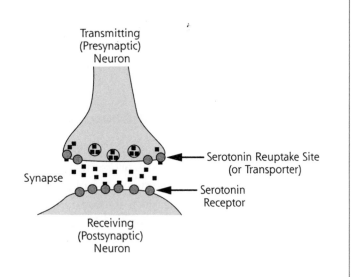

Treatment with anti-
depressants has become
the standard of care for
major depression.

in tyramine (found in certain kinds of wine and aged cheese), then the level of tyramine in the blood can increase (because it can no longer be broken down by monoamine oxidase, which has been put out of commission). Increased tyramine can raise blood pressure to dangerous levels. MAOIs react with foods containing monosodium glutamate (MSG), which is widely used in homes and restaurants to enhance food flavor, resulting in increased tyramine levels. MAOIs can also react with certain over-the-counter medications, with the same effect. In view of these possible adverse reactions, persons taking MAOIs have to be careful what they ingest. (Note: The list above is not exhaustive. Patients taking MAOIs should obtain from their doctor a complete list of foods to avoid.) Though for some patients[1] MAOIs can be the most effective type of drug available in their particular case, they are not usually used as a first line of treatment for depression since a strict diet may be hard for some depressed people to follow religiously. An MAOI patch with fewer side effects is under development but not yet approved by the FDA. Thus far it has only been developed for selegiline, an MAOI not commonly used for treatment of depression.

Tricyclics—amitriptyline, nortriptyline, imipramine, desipramine, doxepine, maprotiline, amoxapine, and clomipramine—tend to overlap several of the classes of drugs described above. Side effects limit their use today because safer drugs are available. However, because of their relatively low cost (especially amitriptyline) tricyclic antidepressants are still used by some people who are financially strapped and without insurance to pay for medication. This category of antidepressants is highly toxic when taken in overdose and used to be a common method of suicide. Newer antidepressants such as SSRIs are not nearly as dangerous if overdosed, which is one reason why they are prescribed so widely today.

Are Antidepressants Effective?

Clinical research studies spanning nearly fifty years have demonstrated that antidepressant drugs are safe and effective treatments for depression, compared to placebo (a sugar pill).[2] Given the risk of suicide associated with depression, treatment with these drugs has become the standard of care for all persons with major depression.[3]

Antidepressants are very effective, despite a highly publicized study that appeared in 2000 in the *Journal of Clinical Psychopharmacology*.[4] Psychiatrist Arif Khan reported that when he analyzed the results of fifty-two studies contained in the FDA's database he found that in only 48 percent of these studies was an antidepressant superior to a sugar pill. Drug companies usually only publish in medical journals the results of those studies with positive results, but the FDA requires that they provide information on all research done to test drugs, so Khan's study of the public record covered a more thorough sample.

Many people in the media interpreted Dr. Khan's results to mean that antidepressants are on average no more effective than placebo and, by implication, that antidepressants really don't work, but that is not true. One must consider how these studies are done and what their results mean in order to understand why—despite such reports—antidepressants are effective in treating more severe depressions over the long term. For one thing, not all depression is the same. Diagnosing depression is not like diagnosing high blood pressure, which can be independently measured. If the blood pressure is above a certain number, a diagnosis of hypertension is made—objectively and verifiably.

As we said earlier, the word *depression* can be used to describe brief, fluctuating periods of bad mood and sadness or it can describe a severe, life-threatening disorder with a 15 percent lifetime mortality rate. Consequently, two persons who are depressed may have very different underlying biological conditions.

Most people who are recruited into depression studies have milder forms of depression. These people typically are not depressed enough to be hospitalized, are functioning well enough to come in for clinic visits, and comply with the study medication. They are never suicidal. They are also otherwise generally physically healthy, as those with severe medical illness or substance abuse that would complicate their depressions are typically excluded from clinical trials. Thus the studies to which Dr. Khan refers in his article involved relatively highly functioning people with mild to moderate uncomplicated depression.

Length of the study also seems to make a difference. The studies that Dr. Khan referred to were carried out for a period of four to eight weeks at most. The "placebo response" (positive response even though only taking sugar pills) is very common among people with mild to moderate depression and typically lasts about eight to twelve weeks. When subjects are followed for longer than that, however, those receiving placebo are much more likely to relapse than those taking antidepressants (as the placebo effect wears off). Antidepressants prove their worth over the long term.

Many people in the media interpreted these results to mean that antidepressants are on average no more effective than placebo and, by implication, that antidepressants really don't work, but that is not true.

Finally, when people are involved in a "double blind" clinical trial to test the effects of an antidepressant versus placebo, they get a lot of attention whether they take the actual drug or the placebo because the clinical staff doesn't know whether a particular subject is on the active drug or the sugar pill. (These studies are called double blind because neither the patient nor the staff knows which patient is receiving the drug being tested versus the placebo.) Another reason subjects receive so much attention is because an enormous effort is often required to keep them in the study and ensure that they take their pills. Thus, study participants usually receive an inordinate amount of monitoring, social support, encouragement, and attention to their worries or concerns.

Of course receiving attention and support and feeling cared for often result in the improvement of a person's depression. Indeed, supportive therapy and encouragement is often the treatment of choice for mild depression. As a result, whether the subjects are taking an active drug or a placebo, the chances of their mild to moderate depression improving just because of the attention they receive in the clinical trial is very high. This "compassion effect" increases the chance of improvement on the placebo—especially in mild depression. Thus, it is not at all surprising to see that many studies find there is little difference between taking a placebo or an antidepressant.

The situation is far different for severe complicated depressions, for subjects during long-term follow-up, or for people unlikely to get the kind of attention that subjects may receive in a clinical trial. Contrary to Dr. Khan's conclusion, ours would be that it is impressive that 52 percent of such studies actually do show a benefit of the antidepressant over the sugar pill, considering all the factors supporting short-term improvement for those in the studies with mild depression.

Antidepressants work. They are effective in the vast majority of patients with clinical depression. It may take time to find the right antidepressant for a person's particular biological makeup, but these drugs are much more effective than sugar pills or no treatment at all. The bottom line is that for three out of four depressed people, antidepressants help to relieve depression, especially when combined with psychotherapy. Less than one in ten depressed people truly have treatment-resistant depression, which persists regardless of treatment with medications (or combinations of medication), psychotherapy, or both. Even many of those with treatment-resistant depression, however, can be treated with electroconvulsive therapy (see chapter 10) and can learn to live a meaningful and quality life, especially with the help of the Lord, caring friends, and good professional treatment.

Factors Involved in Choosing an Antidepressant

Most antidepressants are similar in the speed with which they work and in their short-term and long-term effectiveness in relieving depression. An exception to this rule is in the case of severe biological depression (sometimes called endogenous or melancholic depression) that typically requires hospitalization. There is some evidence that SSRIs such as fluoxetine do not work as well as tricyclic antidepressants such as nortriptyline or desipramine in these kinds of depression. The evidence for this, however, is limited to only a few studies.

Sometimes the effectiveness of an antidepressant can be predicted by the response of other blood relatives. If a depressed person's family member has successfully responded to an antidepressant, this increases the likelihood that the depressed person will respond in a similar way, due to the similarity in biological makeup and expected biochemical response to the antidepressant.

In most cases, the choice of antidepressant is based more on finances and potential side effects. Particularly for those on a limited budget or without insurance coverage, cost can be a significant factor. For example, 100 tablets of 100 mg generic amitriptyline costs between $3.53 and $19.95, compared to $214.46 for 100 tablets of 20 mg paroxetine (not available in generic), $221.37 for 100 tablets of 50 mg sertraline (not available in generic), or $250.14 for 100 capsules of 20 mg fluoxetine (generic fluoxetine is now available and less expensive, i.e., $124.00).[5]

Potential side effects are something else the doctor will consider, often trying to match side effects to the depressed person's symptoms (for example, insomnia might be treated with an antidepressant that has sedation as a side effect). Each antidepressant has a different constellation of possible side effects, so it's important to know the unique side effects associated with each. Not every person will experience side effects to these medications, and perhaps the majority will experience no side effects at all or only very minor ones (especially with the newer antidepressants). Side effects do tend to increase with a person's age (especially for tricyclics), requiring that antidepressants be prescribed with special caution for those over age sixty-five.

If a depressed person's family member has successfully responded to an antidepressant, this increases the likelihood that the depressed person will respond in a similar way.

Side Effects of Antidepressants

All powerful drugs, including antidepressants, have side effects. Some drugs have many; some have few. Usually, the more recent a medication may be, the less side effects it will have, but no one can know in advance which side effect(s) will occur in a particular case. The good news is that the side effects of most antidepressants are minor compared to the value of their therapeutic effect on depression. When side effects do occur, they are often short-lived, as the person's body accommodates to them.[6] Here are some common side effects:

Sedation. Some antidepressants cause people to feel sleepy and help to improve sleep. This is especially true for tricyclics such as amitriptyline, nortriptyline, and doxepine. Nontricyclics that cause sedation include nefazadone, trazodone, and mirtazapine. If the person has difficulty sleeping or is feeling anxious and agitated, then this side effect is very helpful. Sometimes, however, the sleepiness lasts into the daytime and causes problems at work, in school, while driving, or when interacting with others, thus impairing function. If a depressed person is sleeping too much (hypersomnia), then these medications may worsen the problem. Sedation with most antidepressants tends to be time-limited, and continued use of the medication over several weeks will allow the body to get used to it.

Insomnia. Some antidepressants interfere with sleep, or at least do so until the body gets used to the medication. These activating antidepressants include tricyclic antidepressants such as imipramine and desipramine and SSRIs such as fluoxetine, paroxetine, and sertraline, especially at higher doses. Bupropion is perhaps the most stimulating of all (being structurally related to amphetamine) and should be taken no later than about two o'clock in the afternoon or it will impair sleep. Of course, if a person is experiencing lethargy, fatigue, and excessive sleeping because of depression, then bupropion may be very helpful in counteracting this.

Dry mouth and constipation. Some tricyclic antidepressants, including amitriptyline and nortriptyline, have anticholinergic effects that tend to reduce production of saliva, causing dry mouth. They also may slow up peristalsis in the colon (resulting in constipation). Bupropion may also cause dry mouth and constipation through a mechanism that is not entirely clear, though it is not the same as that which occurs with tricyclic antidepressants. Dry mouth can result in tooth decay and cavities especially in older adults. Constipation can be a real problem for those who are already predisposed to this condition due to reduced bowel motility and low fiber and fluid intake.

Drop in blood pressure. Because of effects on nerves that encircle blood vessels, older tricyclic antidepressants such as amitriptyline, imipramine, or doxepine and MAOIs such as phenelzine and tranylcypromine can cause a drop in blood pressure when a person stands up from a reclining or sitting position. Most of the time this is accompanied by temporary lightheadedness, which quickly passes. In older adults with heart problems, people taking other medications that affect blood pressure, or those who are dehydrated because of inadequate fluid intake, this drop in blood pressure may cause a fall or, in very rare cases, even bring on a heart attack or stroke.

Dizziness. Dizziness can be a direct effect of an antidepressant on the balance mechanism in the inner ear or it can be an indirect effect due to a drop in blood pressure. Older adults whose balance and equilibrium may already be compromised due to other medical problems are more likely to be affected by this problem than are younger persons with more reserve. Although this symptom tends to be time-limited, it may persist for months in certain individuals. SSRIs are occasionally associated with dizziness, but this is uncommon.

Increase in blood pressure. The newer antidepressants mirtazapine and venlafaxine may cause an increase in blood pressure especially at higher doses and especially in older adults who may already be predisposed to hypertension. If this occurs, discontinuation of these medications will return the blood pressure to its previous level. Alternatively, if the person is taking antihypertensive medication, increasing the dose of that medicine may allow the person to continue taking one of these antidepressants if it is particularly effective in relieving depression. This is an option the patient should only pursue with the doctor's advice and consent.

Effects on heart conduction. Tricyclic antidepressants may interfere with the conduction of nerve impulses in the heart and therefore cause heart block (where the heart beats much slower than usual) or arrhythmia (irregular or very fast heartbeats). This is much less common with the SSRIs and newer antidepressants.

Nausea and GI upset. Many people experience nausea and/or diarrhea soon after beginning an antidepressant. Sertraline has this effect as do most of the other SSRIs, venlafaxine, and bupropion. This side effect diminishes over time. In some people, however, chronic diarrhea or loose stools becomes a problem that needs to be managed. If diarrhea becomes chronic, then combining an SSRI with a constipating tricyclic antidepressant may help to diminish GI upset and improve antidepressant response.

Sexual side effects. While loss of sexual desire is a common symptom of depression, and treatment of depression may relieve this symptom, certain antidepressants are known to interfere with sexual interest and function even after depression has lifted (causing erectile dysfunction or decreased ability to reach orgasm or ejaculate). This is particularly true for the SSRIs, all of which have this disturbing effect to some extent. Some antidepressants, such as bupropion and trazodone, may actually increase sexual interest and performance. These latter drugs are sometimes used in combination with other antidepressants (such as SSRIs) to counteract their sexual side effects (especially if the depression is under control but sexual side effects are disturbing the patient's quality of life). Mirtazapine is a newer antidepressant that has not been associated with sexual problems in controlled clinical trials.

Weight gain. Many antidepressants cause weight gain, especially the tricyclic antidepressants and most antidepressants that have sedation as a side effect. These medications affect histamine receptors in the brain that make one feel sleepy or hungry. The nontricyclic antidepressant mirtazapine also stimulates appetite (and can result in weight gain). If a depressed person has lost weight due to a loss of appetite, then these medications may facilitate weight gain. On the other hand, if a person has been overeating and gaining weight as a symptom of depression, such an antidepressant may worsen the problem. The SSRIs are less likely to cause weight gain, as are venlafaxine and bupropion. Bupropion, in fact, may be useful for those who are overweight or wishing to lose weight. In most people, the effects of antidepressants on weight tend to stabilize over time.

Restlessness or jitteriness. Antidepressants such as fluoxetine and other SSRIs, bupropion, or desipramine may be associated with initial side effects such as jitteriness, agitation, or restless anxiety. This can be a particular problem in depressed patients who are already anxious or agitated. SSRIs have also been associated with a phenomenon called akithesia, which is seen in some persons taking major tranquilizers such as haloperidol or Thorazine. This is a kind of internal, under-the-skin restlessness. It is a relatively rare side effect but disturbing when it occurs.

Reported Side-Effects of Antidepressants

Drug	Sedation, Sleepiness	Dry Mouth, Constipation	Drop in BP* on Standing	Nausea, GI* Upset	Decreased Sex Drive	Weight Gain
Tricyclics						
Amitriptyline	+ + + +	+ + + +	+ + + +	–	+/–	+ + +
Doxepine	+ + + +	+ + + +	+ + + +	–	+/–	+ + +
Nortriptyline	+ + +	+ + +	+ + +	–	+/–	+ + +
Desipramine	+ +	+ +	+ + +	–	+/–	+ +
SSRIs*						
Fluoxetine	+	+	+	+ +	+ + +	+/–
Sertraline	+	+	+	+ +	+ + +	+/–
Paroxetine	+	+ +	+	+ +	+ + +	+/–
Citalopram	+	+	+	+ +	+ + +	+/–
Escitalopram	+	+	+	+ +	+ + +	+/–
Others						
Venlafaxine	+	+	+	+	+ +	+/–
Mirtazapine	+ + +	+	+	+ +	+	+ + +
Bupropion	+	+	+	+ +	–	–
Trazodone	+ + + +	+	+ + +	–	–	+/–
Nefazadone	+ + +	+	+	+/–	–	+/–
MAO* inhibitors						
Phenelzine	+	+ +	+ + +	+/–	+	+/–
Tranylcypromine	+	+	+ + +	+/–	+	+/–
Mood Stabilizers						
Lithium carbonate	+ +	–	–	–	–	+ + +
Valproic acid	+ +	–	–	–	–	+ + +
Stimulants						
Methylphenidate	–	–	–	+/–	–	–

*BP = blood pressure
GI = gastrointestinal
MAO = monoamine oxidase
SSRI = selective serotonin reuptake inhibitor

Scale: Four plus signs = strong
Three plus signs = moderate
Two plus signs = weak
One plus sign = negligible
Negative sign = none

Minimizing Side Effects

Gradually increasing the dose of anti-depressants allows the body to accommodate to any side effects.

Most of the side effects of antidepressants can be minimized. First, the initial dose should be low. For example, fluoxetine may be started out at a dose of 5 mg to 7.5 mg per day (total of one 20 mg capsule every three to four days), sertraline at a dose of 12.5 mg per day (one-quarter of a 50 mg tablet per day), or bupropion at one 75 mg tablet per day. Ordinarily, these low doses are doubled each week until the target dose is reached.[7] Gradually increasing the dose allows the body to accommodate to any side effects. This means, however, that a therapeutic dose (a daily dose large enough to really help the patient) may not be reached for nearly a month. If depression is relatively mild in severity, this may not be a problem. If depression is severe, the dose will have to be increased more rapidly and the patient will simply have to learn to tolerate the side effects, especially if they are not severe.

Medication should also be taken at a time during the day when side effects will be least noticed and least likely to interfere with functioning. For example, if paroxetine causes sedation, then it should be taken at bedtime. If morning drowsiness is still a problem, then the medication should be taken after supper to give it as much time as possible to allow the level of the drug in the blood to decrease before morning. If a medication causes nausea or dizziness, then taking it at bedtime will minimize these, and by the next morning the symptom should have worn off. Note that in terms of effectiveness, it makes absolutely no difference what time of the day a medication is taken, so side effects are the only factor that should determine this. Taking medication with food may diminish side effects due to a more gradual absorption into the system and less gastrointestinal irritation. Further, certain combinations of antidepressant medications may reduce side effects to one or the other drug. A psychiatrist or physician with experience prescribing antidepressants is most likely to know which combinations are best for which side effects.

Resistance to Taking Medication

Antidepressants help to relieve the suffering of depression faster than any treatment except ECT (see chapter 10). They work much more quickly than psychotherapy and can lift depressed persons up to a point where they can at least work with a therapist in changing thoughts, behaviors, or attitudes. For Christians, antidepressants may help to break the paralysis that prevents a person from praying, reading the Bible, or getting out to church. Thus, antidepressants can at least start you on the road to recovery by helping you function to the point where you can start working on your unique stressors in order to achieve more permanent and lasting gains. Antidepressants can truly be lifesaving, and for some depressed persons with a strong biological component to their depression, they are necessary and unavoidable.

Despite these benefits, however, both Christians and non-Christians typically resist taking antidepressants. Based on a 1986 Roper poll, only 12 percent of Americans indicated they would be willing to take medication for depression.[8] Instead, 78 percent stated they would rather live with the depression until it passed than resort to medication. Things have changed since 1986, as an ABC News poll conducted in April 2000 found that 28 percent of Americans would be willing to take antidepressants for an extended period even if they were informed that there were no safety studies on long-term use.[9]

Why is it that most people are not willing to take antidepressants? Some people are reluctant to take them because of what they have observed in others or what they have been told about medication. They may fear that such treatments will turn them into zombies or put them into a fog. No doubt there are many horror stories to support this fear.

Some patients have been misdiagnosed and treated with the wrong medication or at the wrong dose. The person reporting the story may have mixed up the mental disorder or diagnosis; instead of depression, someone might be reporting a story about a person with schizophrenia, bipolar disorder, or a severe personality disorder. People with psychotic depression may be so seriously ill that they require heavily sedating drugs just to function outside of a hospital setting or to insure their safety and the safety of others. There is a fine balance between undertreatment, adequate treatment, and overtreatment, and some doctors without extensive training and experience (and even some with it) sometimes overshoot the mark. As noted earlier, every person has a different biochemical makeup and will respond in a unique way to a particular medication or dose of medication. Antidepressants are not like antibiotics or antihypertensives that have specific doses and predictable responses in people.

Some people fear they will become dependent on these drugs to feel normal. Also, they don't want to have to rely on medications, which are a constant reminder that they are somehow inadequate, different, abnormal, or defective. Others resist antidepressant medication because they don't know how it works or why they might need it. In this case, their reservation is based on lack of adequate information about the causes of

Antidepressants help to relieve the suffering of depression faster than any treatment except ECT.

Doctors sometimes don't inform patients that after starting antidepressant medication it may take several weeks or months before they start feeling better.

depression and how these drugs work to relieve underlying chemical imbalances.

Doctors sometimes don't inform patients that after starting antidepressant medication it may take several weeks or months before they start feeling better. Furthermore, because each person has such a unique physical makeup, no one can tell ahead of time what drug or combination of drugs will help to improve an individual's symptoms. This last point is crucial because medical doctors (and sometimes psychiatrists) often don't mention this, and patients may be reluctant to tell the doctor that whatever they've been given is not really working. People sometimes feel the doctor is using them as a guinea pig simply because the doctor failed to mention that no one can know in advance what drug, combination of drugs, or dosage is going to work for a particular person. Patients need to know from the outset that finding the right antidepressant medication for their particular case may involve a lot of trial and error.

Some people believe that medication for the treatment of depressive disorders is overprescribed. A 2002 report to the *Journal of the American Medical Association* found that the proportion of persons receiving treatment for depression increased more than threefold in the ten-year period between 1987 and 1997.[10] Based on information collected on over 65,000 medical patients, the researchers found that treatment increased from 0.73 per 100 persons in 1987 to 2.33 per 100 persons in 1997. Of particular interest was the finding that the proportion of treated individuals who used antidepressant medications increased from 37.3 percent to 74.5 percent, whereas the proportion receiving psychotherapy decreased from 71.1 percent to 60.2 percent. The proportion of patients who were treated by general medical physicians (vs. psychologist or social worker) increased from 68.9 percent to 87.3 percent.

While the increasing treatment of depression by physicians was attributed in part to less stigma associated with having depression, patients being more willing to receive treatment, and treatment having fewer side effects, the authors also noted that there was increased pressure placed by managed care organizations on physicians to treat with medication rather than refer patients for more expensive, time-consuming psychotherapy. Unfortunately, many primary care physicians have neither the training nor the interest necessary to treat and manage persons with serious depression.

Doctors are not alone to blame for overprescribing. Patients, too, would rather simply take a pill than go to therapy where they might have to expend a great deal of energy in order to learn new ways of thinking and behaving. Apparently if some patients don't receive a prescription when they leave the doctor's office, they somehow feel unfulfilled. Doctors want to meet patients' expectations. Furthermore, since time is limited, prescribing medication is a much faster way of dealing with the problem, compared to taking time to listen or trying to understand the reasons for the patient's depression. Because everyone is looking for a quick fix (both doctors who don't have time to talk with patients and patients who don't want to take the time or make the effort necessary to change), it is not surprising that long-term solutions to depression are being sought with decreasing frequency.

Indeed, the whole experience can seem like a maze for chronically depressed people who have been receiving treatment for an extended period. Doctors may switch medication or add medication to augment treatment without really giving the first medication a chance to take effect. Patients sometimes stop taking their medication because they are unwilling to deal with side effects that may be only temporary. This is made worse when doctors have not provided adequate education about possible side effects and the likelihood that they will diminish with time. The doctor may not tell the patient when to expect improvement, so the patient may stop taking a drug before it has had time to work.

Some patients report they have been on quite a few different drugs that range from antidepressants to minor tranquilizers to antipsychotics. There is concern about how these drugs might be affecting body chemistry. When drugs are piled one on top of another, just trying to keep track of it all can seem overwhelming.

While some of these concerns are valid, many are unfounded. Antidepressant drugs used today have typically undergone extensive testing in humans and animals over a period of decades to determine their effectiveness and side effects. Since the 1960s, no antidepressant has had to be taken off the market because of long-term side effects, despite the fact that hundreds of thousands of people have been taking these drugs for years. A few years ago there was concern that fluoxetine increased the risk of suicide. However, further study found fluoxetine to be no different than other antidepressant drugs in this regard (and the suicide rate in depressed people who did not receive antidepressant treatment was vastly higher by comparison).

Some people might be better off if they could flush all of the drugs out of their system and then be reevaluated. But this seldom happens, primarily because if someone with depression is not doing well, doctors are reluctant to stop medication for fear the patient's condition might

Antidepressant drugs used today have typically undergone extensive testing in humans and animals over a period of decades to determine their effectiveness and side effects.

Switching to another antidepressant, either within the same medication class or to a different class, is usually effective in returning responsiveness.

abruptly worsen, which might lead to suicide. If such a cleansing could take place in a supervised setting such as a hospital, then doctors would be more likely to try it. Unfortunately, in this day of managed care only brief hospitalizations are permitted. Such short stays are not adequate to wash out drugs and then monitor the response—which may take a long time to stabilize.

The basic issue for both patients and physicians is communication. People who can be helped by medication need to have straight talk from their doctors. They also need to question the doctor when he or she prescribes medication.[11] However, when people are seriously depressed, they don't always have the ability to think clearly enough to ask the right questions, and most don't have a knowledgeable person to be an advocate for them. Doctors seem godlike, so it is tempting to accept what they say as gospel. Yet it is in every patient's best interests to find out as much as possible about any drugs prescribed, whether by consulting the *Physician's Desk Reference* or another printed source or via computer on the internet, where information can be obtained easily by typing in the drug's brand name or generic name or by simply typing the words *medication* and *depression*.

Remember, however, just because a side effect is listed in the *Physician's Desk Reference* or on the internet doesn't necessarily mean that a patient will experience this side effect or that if they do have a symptom listed that it is necessarily a side effect of the antidepressant being taken. Both the patient and the physician must work together to determine whether a symptom is a side effect of an antidepressant, is due to another medication, or is a new symptom due to another medical or psychiatric condition.

When an Antidepressant Stops Working

It is not uncommon for antidepressants to stop working after a person has been taking them for several years. This is especially true if ongoing environmental stress, internal psychological conflict, or bad decisions are continuing to deplete the neurotransmitters that maintain normal mood. It may even occur as a result of unusual stress or disorder in one's spiritual life. In any case, when a medication has lost its effect, physicians can do several things to restore drug effectiveness.

Switching to another antidepressant, either within the same medication class or to a different class, is usually effective in returning responsiveness. For example, if a person has been on fluoxetine, sertraline, or paroxetine for several years and it is no longer working, he or she may respond well to venlafaxine or mirtazapine. Often the person will gain a benefit from the new medication that lasts for months or even years. After some time he or she could be switched back to the original antidepressant and it might work again. If switching to another medication in the same drug class does not work, then the doctor should try a medication in another drug class. For example, if the venlafaxine or mirtazapine does not help, then bupropion or possibly nortriptyline might be effective. If neither of these work, then an MAOI (such as phenelzine or tranylcypromine) might do so. One of these drugs will almost always work if prescribed and taken at an adequate dose for an adequate period of time.

Sometimes combinations of drugs may work when either drug alone does not.

Sometimes combinations of drugs may work when either drug alone does not. For example, a tricyclic antidepressant such as nortriptyline may be combined with an SSRI such as fluoxetine. The dose of nortriptyline can be lower than ordinarily prescribed alone, sometimes reducing side effects. An SSRI can be used in combination with trazodone (for those with sleep disturbance) or sometimes bupropion (for those with sexual side effects). Such a combination may also boost antidepressant effectiveness. By contrast, certain antidepressant drug combinations (such as an MAO inhibitor and an SSRI) may have disastrous consequences (hypertensive crisis or serotonin syndrome), so combinations of antidepressants should only be prescribed by physicians who are familiar with this approach.

Antidepressant effects may also be boosted by a strategy called augmentation, in which the doctor may add small doses of lithium or thyroid hormone to the antidepressant regimen. This strategy has been used for over twenty-five years with good results in some patients. Thus, when a person with a history of numerous recurrent depressions has chosen to remain on lifelong antidepressant drug therapy, there are many things a physician can do to help the patient maintain a response (especially if they are done in concert with addressing situational, internal, and interpersonal stressors in his or her life).

Spiritual Issues Related to Antidepressants

One fundamental question for believers is: "What does the Bible have to say about the use of antidepressants?" The answer: nothing.

What does the Bible have to say about the use of antidepressants? Nothing.

We realize that some Christian counselors and pastors teach that using anything other than the Bible, faith, and the Holy Spirit's power to overcome life's difficulties, including depression, is wrong. If depression were purely an issue of the spirit, we would have no problem with this assertion, as in a spiritual sense these three components are all believers need for life and godliness. However, since depression is a whole-person issue, it is rarely a purely spiritual matter. What affects us spiritually affects us psychologically, sociologically, and physically, and vice versa.

We expect that those who promote the idea that depression should only be treated by the Bible and faith have never spent time with Christians struggling with serious psychiatric disorders, whether in a psychiatric ward or outside. Had they done so, they might not be so quick to deny the value of pharmacological intervention in some cases.

Having said that, however, let us repeat that without doubt clinical depression *is* a spiritual issue (as well as a physical, sociological, and psychological issue). Therefore, those who are followers of Christ would be wise to consider these four questions:

1. *What is God trying to say to you through your depression?* This is the primary question because if you believe God may be trying to say *anything* to you through your depression, then the spiritual issue related to taking a pill to alleviate the pain is whether you will then be able to hear perhaps the most important divine message you'll ever receive. Some Christian counselors might say that on medication you will be desensitized to God's Spirit, deaf to his voice. However, if you are clinically depressed you may *never be able* to discern God's voice until you find the right medication at the right dose to restore your equilibrium. Instead, you may hear (and possibly respond to) many other voices.

In my spiritual self, I (DB) want to hear whatever God wishes to say. While writing these words, I am in a tent in the Colorado Rockies at nearly 10,000 feet elevation, surrounded by towering mountains that proclaim the awesome majesty and power of God. Without the medication I take, I would not be able to hear what God wants to say to me. I wish, how I wish, that I didn't need pills to keep me from the pit, but my struggle has lasted so long that this is now my reality. In other words, thanks to the right medication at the right dose, I am enabled to be who I really want to be in a physical *and* spiritual sense. Since this is consistent with my understanding of God's will for me, I fail to see how it could possibly be anathema in his eyes.

2. Does your taking medication imply that you don't believe that the Bible, faith, and the Holy Spirit's empowerment are enough in matters of the heart? Not necessarily. For example, anyone who has been clinically depressed knows how hard it is to concentrate on *anything*, much less on understanding and applying biblical texts and principles to the practical issues of our lives. Taking medication so that your normal mental functions return may actually pave the way for better understanding and application of God's truths to your life on a day-to-day basis. Nor does taking medication imply that you are substituting a false god (medicine) and its truth for the real God and his truth. Medicine in this case can facilitate deeper understanding of God's Word, a more cogent perception of faith, and a more coherent appropriation of the power of his Spirit. Those who hope in medicine will find only disappointment in the end; those who hope in God and use medicine as a means to fulfilling his purposes quite often will find the healing they need.

3. Do you want your medication to mask the underlying issues that have contributed to your depression, thereby relieving you of some degree of responsibility for dealing with them? An answer of "yes" to this question should be a red flag for any believer. We are called to know the truth that will set us free to be and become what God wants us to be.

4. Finally, are you willing to allow antidepressant medication to clear your mind so you can face your issues with the help of a counselor or trusted friend? Responding "yes" to this question means that you will need to find someone who will faithfully help you discover and resolve matters that need closure, discern issues in your actions or thinking that may be blocking your progress in the Christian life, and develop new strategies and behaviors that will honor your Lord, advancing you toward maturity in him.

The bottom line in terms of spiritual issues related to antidepressants is this: If you are not severely depressed and are convinced that using antidepressants would be wrong and that without antidepressants you will be enabled to better know God, and his Son, then you should consider, with the advice and consent of your family, friends, and spiritual advisors, finding a mature Christian counselor who can help you explore and try to resolve the various factors that contribute to your depression without the use of medications. If you believe the use of antidepressants will enable you to function more normally and may increase your ability to ponder the deeper issues of the heart that may be related to your depression, then you should seek the help of both a Christian physician and a Christian counselor (or counselors) who are willing and

Those who hope in medicine will find only disappointment in the end; those who hope in God and use medicine as a means to fulfilling his purposes quite often will find the healing they need.

In the end, whatever you decide, the main thing worth taking from your experience with depression is the deeper knowledge that real hope is only found in one place—an ever-deepening relationship with Christ, who understands the depths of our pain and died to heal it all.

able to help you press on toward the mark of the higher calling of God in Christ Jesus (see Phil. 3:12–14). In the end, whatever you decide, the main thing worth taking from your experience with depression is the deeper knowledge that real hope is only found in one place—an ever-deepening relationship with Christ, who understands the depths of our pain and died to heal it all.

What Antidepressants Can't Do

Antidepressants are extremely helpful in relieving depression. However, they are not wonder drugs that permanently and miraculously cure depression. More than just medication is usually required to achieve complete and lasting healing (wholeness). Antidepressants cannot make up for habitual bad decisions, insensitivity to the needs of others, or spiritually wayward behavior. If psychosocial stressors, self-destructive actions, or self-defeating thinking continue, the restorative effects of antidepressants will be diminished. Thus, it is extremely important to understand what is at the root of the depression and try to deal with that. Antidepressants do not excuse a person from changing when change is necessary. They only give people a reprieve for a little while in order to get their lives back together. If that time is wasted, then depression will likely return sooner or later, perhaps more brutal than before.

This is true not only for those with situational, spiritual, or developmental depressions, but also to some extent for persons with primary biological depressions. People with biological depression are especially vulnerable to even small personal misbehaviors or stress-producing decisions that easily precipitate depression (where similar stress would have little or no effect on those without such vulnerability). These people must learn to pay special attention to psychological, social, or spiritual stress that might launch an episode of depression. They seem especially sensitive to the effects of the smallest emotional stress, failure, or loss. The same is true for persons with long-standing tendency to depression due to experiences during childhood or early development, again due to little or no fault of their own. In any case, the responsibility remains ours, whatever our background or stressors, to cease blaming others or outside factors for our depression and to chart a new course toward wholeness that neither happenings nor history can modify. Accepting this responsibility is one of the marks of maturity.

Straight Talk with Your Doctor

Patients and family members need to know what to expect from their physicians, and physicians need to know that everyone is properly informed. Straight talk about the following issues should help all parties concerned to proceed with mutual understanding. Here are some questions to ask and issues to consider:

Are we sure the diagnosis is correct? Many other conditions look like depression but are not. For example, an older adult may be developing dementia, which may appear like depression. Similarly, a younger person may have bipolar disorder and be in the depressed phase. Prescribing an antidepressant may bring on a manic episode and cause a destabilization of the bipolar illness. Depression may be from a side effect or an interaction of medications (prescription or over-the-counter) the patient is already taking.

Depression can be confused with fatigue or loss of energy due to an undiagnosed medical condition, which is why each patient thought to have depression should have a full medical workup. Medical conditions that can cause depression include (alphabetically): AIDS, alcohol abuse, B-12 deficiency, chronic fatigue syndrome, Cushing's disease, epilepsy, head trauma, heart disease, hepatitis, hyperthyroidism, hypothyroidism, infections (bacterial or viral), lupus (SLE), migraine headaches, multiple sclerosis, Parkinson's disease, postpartum physical or emotional changes, postsurgical physical or emotional changes, premenstrual syndrome (PMS), and strokes.

Does this depression need an antidepressant? Many people experience depressed moods that fluctuate from day-to-day but do not last in a sustained manner and are not associated with difficulty sleeping, weight loss, or other significant depressive symptoms. These people do not need antidepressant therapy but rather counseling to help them better deal with their day-to-day problems. Similarly, if there are long-term character or personality factors that underlie a depression, then psychotherapy is more likely to help than medication.

Is anything more than an antidepressant medication needed? Antidepressants by themselves are often not sufficient to treat a depression. Usually some kind of support, counseling, or psychotherapy is also necessary, since there are almost always problems coping with life situations that underlie or at least contribute to the depression. An antidepressant will not change difficult life circumstances that must be adapted to nor

The responsibility remains ours, whatever our background or stressors, to cease blaming others or outside factors for our depression and to chart a new course toward wholeness that neither happenings nor history can modify.

will it enable a person to make better decisions if he or she habitually makes poor ones. Psychotherapy is necessary to address these issues.

How might the antidepressant interact with other medications? Antidepressants can interact with and interfere with other prescription or over-the-counter medications the patient is taking. For example, Paxil or Prozac can interfere with the breakdown of the blood-thinner Warfarin or Coumadin, requiring that the dose of the blood-thinner be adjusted in order to keep the patient from experiencing a stroke or serious bleeding.

Is the medication affordable? Most of the newer antidepressants cost between $2.00 and $3.00 per pill. If patients are on a limited income or don't have insurance, they may not be able to afford the medication and therefore will not be able to comply with the prescription. Since the doctor might not ask, patients should request that generic drugs be prescribed when they are available, as long as these drugs are identical to brand name drugs in their effect on depression. Most people can afford generic drugs even if they don't have health insurance, and many health insurance plans have a lower co-pay when generics are purchased.

What are the possible side effects? Patients should ask about what side effects to expect from the antidepressant and how long to expect them. They need to know exactly what to do and whom to call if they start having side effects. They should understand what side effects should prompt the patient to stop taking the medication immediately. They should also understand which side effects they should try to tolerate because they will usually resolve with time. They should become informed on how to minimize side effects.

How should the medication be taken? All antidepressant medication should be started at a low dose and gradually increased. The patient should understand how and when to increase the medication, whether to take the medicine at night or in the morning, and whether to take it with food or on an empty stomach. These instructions should be provided by the doctor and also be included when the pharmacist delivers the medication. The patient needs to know what food, drink, and activities must be avoided. Others who may be monitoring the patient's use of the medication also need to understand what has been said.

How long will it be before improvement should be seen? An antidepressant must be taken at the full therapeutic dose for a minimum of six weeks before a conclusion can be reached that the medicine is not working. Patients need to know that they might feel worse (due to side effects from the medication as their body gets used to it) before they feel better. They should be informed that it is unlikely that they will feel better before they have taken the medication for at least two or three weeks.

How will changes in the antidepressant's dosage be handled? Patients should call their doctor before they reduce the medication's dose or stop taking it. Such dosage reduction or drug discontinuation can result in an unpleasant withdrawal reaction and may contribute to a relapse into depression. For the same reason, patients should also be careful to refill their prescriptions in a timely way so they won't run out.

When will it be possible to discontinue taking the medication? Patients having their first or second episode of depression should expect to continue taking the antidepressant for at least nine months after they have experienced a full remission of symptoms. Patients who have had three or more episodes of major depression in the past should probably be on lifelong treatment with an antidepressant medication. If depression recurs because medication is discontinued, depressive episodes may become more severe and difficult to control in the future. This is because every episode of recurrent depression may lead to permanent brain changes that increase future vulnerability.

What if the treatment doesn't work? The doctor should acknowledge that no one can know in advance which medication at what dose and for what duration will be most effective for a given patient. In light of this fact, the doctor should communicate that he or she will stick with the patient through each round of trial and error in relation to medications until the right medication and dosage are determined. The patient should not be surprised to hear that while the doctor sees and treats many patients with depression, a time may come when the help of a specialist such as a psychiatrist may be needed in order to find the right drugs or combination of drugs in this particular case. If that time does come, both patient and doctor should view such a referral as the next step in the treatment plan rather than as a failure.

Is the doctor willing to take a team approach to treatment? Since a combination of treatments is more effective for most patients with depression, the doctor should be willing to work with other professional caregivers toward the return of the patient's physical, emotional, and spiritual health. We are convinced that the treatment team's synergistic relationship will prove invaluable to the patient in terms of his or her journey toward joy again.

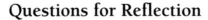

Questions for Reflection

1. What would you include in your list of questions to ask your physician about antidepressant medication?

2. What did you find most helpful about the sketches relating to how antidepressants work?

3. Were you surprised to learn that settling on the right dose of the right antidepressant for treating your depression is a matter of trial and error? In light of this, what would you wish your physician to communicate to you about the process?

4. What do you think is the main reason that many people would resist taking antidepressants?

5. Do you think that more people are depressed these days than in the past or that more people today are willing to seek help?

6. What is your greatest fear in relation to the prospect of taking antidepressants?

7. Which of the spiritual issues related to taking antidepressants seems most important to you?

8. Review the section on straight talk with your doctor. What would you add to this list? What would you leave out?

9. Identify your reasons for being willing to take antidepressants or your reasons for resisting the use of such medications.

CHAPTER 10

Other Treatments for Depression

Taken together, psychotherapy and antidepressants are effective in 75 to 80 percent of clinical depression cases. Sometimes, however, other treatments are needed.

Although there are many alternative treatments for depression, we limit our discussion to other medications (mood stabilizers, antianxiety drugs, and antipsychotic drugs),[1] hospitalization, and less conventional treatments such as electroconvulsive therapy (ECT), estrogen therapy, repetitive transcranial magnet stimulation, and vagus nerve stimulation. We also describe less commonly used Christian therapies including fasting, group prayer and laying on of hands, exorcism, and radical forgiveness with visualization and/or role-playing.

Medications besides Antidepressants

Cathy recently completed her M.B.A., although she could only take one course at a time due to a kidney condition. She has established Cherish, Inc., "a non-profit organization to provide mental health ministry that lifts up Jesus Christ and offers comfort, reassurance, guidance, support, and a sense of belonging through the Christian faith." The following is a condensed version of her testimony, which she wrote especially for inclusion in this book:

"I knew there was something wrong with me the summer before entering high school, when I fell into my first deep depression. Thankfully, this was also about the time I became a Christian. I became moody and lost my ability to laugh. I would rarely speak. My mother was always encouraging me to invite a friend over. But when I did, I just wasn't good company, and it made me feel even worse. Eventually my self-esteem became so low that I would hide in my bedroom and cry, wondering what I had done wrong to be feeling so bad about myself.

"I survived a stormy four years in high school, with my bipolar disorder untreated and unrecognized. I was very unhappy most of the time, plagued by the *if onlys* like: *If only I had more friends, I would be happy. If only I could make the tennis team, I would be happy. If only I could get that hot job at the mall, I would be happy. If only I could please my parents, . . . if only I could make it into the right college.* The list was endless as I lived for the future because the present was so painful. I attributed my emotions to the circumstances of my life, because I lacked the education and insight to call it what it was: depression. Even my highly educated parents were ignorant when it came to my moods.

"During my final year of high school my older sister got me a job at the local fast food restaurant, which was *the* hangout in our small town. My depression lifted as I found validation in a job well done and friendship among my coworkers. Finally, I was able to function with a smile. It wasn't long until my upbeat temperament attracted the new trigger for my roller-coaster emotions—men! Wow—exciting times! New highs—and crashing lows. My relationships were never stable. I knew nothing of drawing boundaries, and my mood swings became more frequent. With each failed relationship I would pull out my journal and romanticize my emotions, pouring out my overwhelming feelings and thoughts in prose and poetry.

"This was how I first became aware that I cycled through depression, as most of my prose was an attempt to deal with and define how I was feeling. My thoughts were dark and morose. Yes, I was off-kilter more often than not. But why? Out of ignorance, I still attributed my depressions to external factors.

"When I was eighteen, before I was to leave for college a friend showed me how to get high. The temporary relief—and control of my mood swings—sure felt good, as did the acceptance from cool people who did drugs. Thus began years of self-medication with marijuana, alcohol, poppers, and an occasional pill that would send me who knows where . . . though to my muddled mind, anywhere but where I was seemed good enough.

"In 1992 'anywhere but here' became a psychiatric ward. After quitting a daily habit of amphetamines and alcohol cold turkey, I experienced a psychotic break from reality. Fearing the food was poisoned, I refused to eat. When the nurse came to give me a shot of Thorazine, she had to bring five others to hold me down. Paranoia had me curled into a fetal position behind my bed until sunrise—hiding from the shadows. This was my hell for five manic, paranoid, sleepless days.

"I may have been clinically out of my mind, but in desperation I called on the Lord Jesus Christ, repeating the only Scripture I knew by heart, 'The Lord's Prayer.' Over and over and over again I repeated it through the night, huddled on the floor. When dawn came I sang the only camp song I could remember: 'It's a happy day, and I thank God for the weather. It's a happy day, and I'm living it for my Lord. It's a happy day, and things are gonna get better, living each day by the promises in God's Word.' In the terror of that room, he was there for me. In the darkness of my mind, he was my light.

"The Lord delivered me from my addictions of amphetamines, alcohol, and marijuana. He also comforted me through Scriptures, including: 'I sought the LORD, and he answered me; he delivered me from all my fears. Those who look to him are radiant; their faces are never covered with shame' (Ps. 34:4–5), and, 'Forgetting what is behind and straining toward what is ahead, I press on toward the goal to win the prize for which God has called me heavenward in Christ Jesus' (Phil. 3:13–14).

"Today when I feel alone and stigmatized, our Lord shares with me his heart full of mercy and compassion! When tears and loneliness seem never-ending, I find a peaceful calm through prayer and worship, and I sing songs of praise when depression and devastation seem thick upon me. Though I have struggled through many hospitalizations recovering from seven breakdowns, none has been as terrifying as the first. No matter how many breakdowns I may experience, I know that he will always walk with me.

"Several years ago I received some life-changing news. One of my blood labs came up abnormal; my lithium level had reached toxicity, and I was in kidney failure [an uncommon complication]. I immediately had to be taken off of lithium, and suddenly I found out what anxiety was all about. Apparently lithium had controlled my anxiety; the newer medications did not. I took Depakote, but it made me confused [another uncommon complication]. I remember having the hardest time just driving down the street to the grocery store and making change at the counter. For a few days I went without food in my house because I forgot I had money in the bank.

"Switching medication was a horrible experience. I went through this for three years, new medication after new medication, adjustment after adjustment. Neurontin did not work—none of the medications worked at the therapeutic level—and now I was under intensive psychiatric care as well as being monitored for my kidneys by a nephrologist. Today I give myself weekly injections to overcome anemia, because my kidneys no longer tell my brain to produce a hormone that stimulates the production of red blood cells. I am somewhat stable on Trileptal (oxcarbazepine), and earlier this year I was able to return to work full-time, but every day is a struggle.

"Yet God used this time of disability for good. No longer do I view myself as a sick person, anticipating the next breakdown and all that it entails. I have found a new foundation for the way I think about my circumstances, my illness, and ultimately my life, and that foundation is a loving relationship with Jesus Christ, who has not only forgiven me of all my sins, but has borne all my shame for me. My reputation now belongs to him; he carries it so that I can move forward, living the life he has placed in me, a life that is no longer my own, for I am bought with the price of his sacrificial love (see 1 Cor. 6:20).

"I now know that my troubles are only momentary compared to the riches of heaven that lie ahead (see 2 Cor. 4:12–18). I know that I am accepted in the Beloved (Eph. 1:6 NASB), that I am an overcomer (1 John 5:4), and that I am spiritually blessed (Eph. 1:3). I know that a Holy Spirit controlled mind leads to life and peace (Rom. 8:6), that I can come boldly to the throne of grace and find help in time of need (Heb. 4:16), and that wisdom to live this challenging life is mine for the asking (James 1:5). I have learned that the lesser ones in the Lord are given special honor (1 Cor. 12:22–23) and that serving the Lord fills me with joy and helps me live a more healthy life. I could go on and on and on, but the best way to find out how God can change a life is to ask him to change yours!"[2]

Sometimes other conditions such as bipolar disorder can be misdiagnosed as clinical depression. Bipolar disorder is a condition related to major depression that does not respond well to drugs classified as antidepressants, particularly if prescribed without medications that stabilize mood. Since in many cases there is a family history of the disease, bipolar disorder may be passed on genetically. The woman whose story you've just read, Cathy, has a sister also afflicted with bipolar disorder. In both cases, the disease's onset occurred during adolescence.

Many patients with bipolar disorder have difficulty managing their treatment. Commonly they stop their medication when their sense of well-being has been restored, which usually results in another cycle of depression and/or mania. The typical disturbing or disruptive behavioral and emotional roller coaster experienced by a person with bipolar disorder is difficult not only for the patient but also for his or her family, friends, and employer (if he or she has been able to work) as well as for medical and other professionals involved.

Lithium can be very effective for preventing recurrent depression, especially if there is a cyclic pattern to the disorder.

Mood Stabilizers

Between 1885 and 1895, two Danish brothers discovered that lithium was capable of reducing the recurrence of depression. It was not until 1949 that lithium became used more widely for the treatment of bipolar disorder, its eventual primary indication. Lithium never did prove to be a very good antidepressant (especially for treatment of depression once an episode got started). However, it can be very effective for preventing recurrent depression, especially if there is a cyclic pattern to the disorder. Lithium is also used to augment or boost the effects of an antidepressant that is not working very well. Lithium has become the mainstay of preventive treatment in bipolar disorder. Studies show that lithium reduces the likelihood of recurrent mania and recurrent depression, which means that some recurrence may occur, but this is surely more tolerable for people with this disorder than having no reprieve at all. Lithium can have a number of side effects (besides the uncommon one that Cathy experienced) including sluggishness, tremors, or weight gain. Without this drug, however, many patients with bipolar disorder experience recurrent episodes of either psychotic mania that completely disrupt their family and work life or severe life-threatening suicidal depression.

Besides lithium, over the past ten years several other mood stabilizers have emerged. They have come from a group of drugs called anticonvulsants for their antiseizure activity. These include carbamazepine (Tegretol) or oxcarbazepine (Trileptal), valproic acid (Depakote), gabapentin (Neurontin), lamotrigine (Lamictal), and topiramate (Topamax). Although usually used to prevent seizures in people with epilepsy, these drugs have been found to stabilize patients with bipolar disorder and to prevent the cycling in and out of recurrent depression. Despite Cathy's negative experience with valproic acid (Depakote), it remains the most commonly used drug for this purpose today, because it has fewer side effects than lithium and appears to be equally effective. Weight gain and hair loss occur in some cases, but these side effects are usually mild. Valproic acid has little effect on relieving an episode of depression once it has begun; therefore, it should be taken prior to the onset of depression.

Because of their rapid effectiveness in relieving distress, antianxiety drugs easily induce dependence and sometimes addiction; these are not antidepressants.

Antianxiety Drugs

In 1960 chlordiazepoxide (Librium) and in 1963 diazepam (Valium) were first marketed for the treatment of anxiety. These drugs and the class of benzodiazepines to which they belong are not antidepressants. They do not relieve an episode of depression. Instead, benzodiazepines rapidly and effectively relieve the severe anxiety that sometimes accompanies depression. A person may experience a reduction in anxiety twenty or thirty minutes after taking the medication. Because of their rapid effectiveness in relieving distress, such drugs easily induce dependence and sometimes addiction. In other words, a person acquires an increasing need for the drug that must be taken in increasing amounts to achieve the same effect. Some short-acting medications such as alprazolam (Xanax) are so difficult to come off of that a person may need to be hospitalized and carefully monitored as the drug is slowly reduced. Longer-acting medication such as diazepam and klonazepam (Klonopin) are easier to come off but may build up in the body and result in oversedation, disequilibrium, memory disturbance, or falls with bone fractures.

These drugs are not antidepressants, since they do not treat the underlying depression. Rather, they temporarily treat the symptom of anxiety just as acetaminophen (Tylenol) may be used to treat a fever that accompanies infection. Tylenol does not treat the infection, only the infection's symptom. The infection itself is usually treated with antibiotics. Anxiety that accompanies depression is a symptom, not the disease itself. The depression should be treated with antidepressants and/or counseling in order for improvement to occur. Over time, benzodiazepines can actually make a depression worse because they are central nervous system depressants with an effect similar to that of alcohol.

Despite this danger, benzodiazepines are especially helpful when severe anxiety or panic attacks accompany depression. People who have both severe anxiety and depression are at increased risk of suicide. So in order to quickly relieve the agitation and distress that may be driving the person toward suicide, benzodiazepines are prescribed for a brief period in order to gain time for the antidepressant drug to start working. Benzodiazepines are also effective in helping people to sleep, although this effect usually wears off with continued use, requiring increasing medication to maintain the benefit. For these reasons, once the antidepressant has started to work, the doctor will slowly reduce and discontinue the dose of antianxiety medication so that dependence does not develop.

Antipsychotic Drugs

In 1952 chlorpromazine (Thorazine) was introduced as the first antipsychotic drug for the treatment of severe agitation and psychosis. By 1954 it was being prescribed widely in state hospitals. In 1958 haloperidol (Haldol) was introduced and soon rivaled Thorazine as the most widely used antipsychotic. Prior to 1954 persons with chronic mental illness, schizophrenia, severe personality disorders, or acute mania had to be institutionalized and sometimes physically restrained from harming themselves or assaulting others. These drugs were heralded as wonder drugs, enabling those who had previously been confined to psychiatric institutions to live independently once again in the community and with their families. However, these medications were accompanied by serious side effects including excessive sedation, muscle stiffness, and shaking (called "Parkinsonism"), and after a period of time strange movements of the lips, tongue, and sometimes extremities (called "tardive dyskinesia"). People taking high doses of these drugs looked like zombies, staring straight ahead, drooling saliva, and walking with stiff movements like Frankenstein in the movies.

Today, thankfully, a new class of safer medications with fewer side effects has largely replaced the older antipsychotics. These drugs, called serotonin-dopamine antagonists, include clozapine (Clozaril, 1990), risperidone (Risperdal), olanzapine (Zyprexa), quetiapine (Seroquel), and most recently, Ziprasidone (Geodon). These drugs may even have some antidepressant effects (although they are still not considered antidepressants). They are used to treat the paranoia, delusions, and hallucinations seen in psychotic depression, in the manic phase of bipolar disorder, and sometimes in cases of severe anxiety. Although high doses may be required initially, they can be reduced gradually once the psychotic illness has been brought under control. The antipsychotics have been very important in enabling people with severe psychiatric conditions to live at home and be cared for by families and loved ones rather than being forced to live in institutions.

Antipsychotics enabled those who had previously been confined to psychiatric institutions to live independently once again in the community and with their families.

Hospitalization

If depression is severe and medical treatments are not working, or a person's physical health is endangered because of severe weight loss, psychotic symptoms, or suicidal behavior, then hospitalization becomes necessary. No one wants to go into the hospital. Patients often plead not

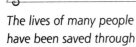

The lives of many people have been saved through acute hospitalization, either voluntarily or involuntarily.

to have to be hospitalized. To them it represents the greatest possible stigmatization. Many times these hospital units are locked, and no one wants to be locked in somewhere, confined with strangers who may be psychotic or otherwise emotionally unstable. This is completely understandable. Hospitalization is truly the treatment of last resort. Nevertheless, the lives of many people have been saved through acute hospitalization,[3] either voluntarily or involuntarily.

Typically, patients will wear their own clothes in the hospital. They may have to share a room with another patient, usually someone with a similar diagnosis. Family members and other persons selected by the patient, such as pastors, are allowed to visit. All patients are expected to participate in the various recreational programs, music therapy, and other activities chosen for their therapeutic value.

Many things can be accomplished during hospitalization that cannot be as efficiently and effectively accomplished outside. First of all, the patient's safety is ensured. Patients in the hospital are carefully monitored to ensure that they don't hurt themselves and also that others don't hurt them. The hospital is the safest place for someone with severe depression, especially if it is associated with psychotic symptoms, emaciation, or suicidal wishes. During a hospitalization, a complete medical and psychiatric evaluation can be completed, including blood tests and other diagnostic procedures as indicated. This evaluation can ascertain the diagnosis and ensure that the appropriate treatment is being administered. A further benefit is that hospitalization removes patients from environments that may have been contributing to their depression. Many patients feel great relief as they move from a chaotic outside world into a secure setting with structured routines.

Another benefit for the hospital patient is that more intensive psychotherapy can be conducted in the hospital than is available to an outpatient. Group or individual therapies can be conducted every day, allowing the cumulative effect of these therapies to build more quickly. Also, family members can be actively involved in both therapy and planning what to do after discharge. Medication changes can be made more rapidly, and new medications can be tried under the constant watchful eye of a hospital staff. Any serious side effects or untoward reactions can be immediately detected and the drugs stopped. Finally, preparations can be made for electroconvulsive therapy, if other treatments fail. Most people remain in the hospital for one to two weeks—seldom longer since most insurance companies will not pay for longer stays. Thus, from the outset patients can be reassured that they will not spend the rest of their lives on the "funny farm," if only because doing so would be too expensive.

Electroconvulsive Therapy

Electroconvulsive therapy (ECT) is extremely effective for major depression, despite the fact that we still don't know exactly how it works.[4] It is likely that ECT changes the levels of neurotransmitters such as serotonin and dopamine in the brain, resetting the levels of these chemicals to a healthier balance. Whatever the exact mechanism, the response rate among depressed persons receiving ECT is 80 to 90 percent, a rate that is greater than that seen with antidepressant medication and/or counseling. Even among people who have failed one or more adequate trials of antidepressant medication, the response rate is still 50 to 60 percent. After a successful course of ECT, however, the depression will likely return within a couple of months unless the person is also placed on antidepressant medication to sustain the response. Following ECT, a person previously completely disabled by depression may be free from further episodes for months or years.

In 1938 ECT was first used to produce convulsions for the treatment of schizophrenia. Within a short time it was being used for the treatment of manic-depressive psychosis. After its discovery, ECT became widely used for the treatment of psychiatric disorders including major depression, psychotic depression, mania, and schizophrenia. ECT was administered indiscriminately and sometimes for the wrong indication, and complications such as bone fractures from uncontrolled seizures were not uncommon. After the mid-1950s, its use began to drop off as medications were discovered to treat these illnesses.

Before the advent of modern medical technology, ECT induced generalized seizures that made a person's entire body convulse, requiring that patients be strapped down and have a bite block placed in their mouths to prevent them from biting their tongues. This was the image presented when Jack Nicholson was forcefully restrained, strapped down on a gurney, and given ECT in the movie *One Flew over the Cuckoo's Nest*. This horrible, barbaric image turned many people against the practice. As a result, some state legislatures outlawed ECT. I (HK) remember visiting the state hospital in Stockton, California, as a nursing student in the late 1970s. The psychiatrist there had been forbidden to treat patients with ECT. Given the lifesaving results he had seen from ECT during his

The hospital is the safest place for someone with severe depression, especially if it is associated with psychotic symptoms, emaciation, or suicidal wishes.

Today ECT is performed with the precision and finesse of a surgical operation. It is extremely safe and extremely effective for major depression.

career, however, the psychiatrist risked his medical credentials by continuing to administer ECT to his patients anyway.

Much of the resistance to ECT has disappeared as the technology has improved and the benefits of treatment have been clearly documented. During the past decade especially, there has been a resurgence of interest in ECT as a treatment for people with drug-resistant depression, those with life-threatening depression (suicidal, severe weight loss, etc.) who cannot wait the time necessary for antidepressant drugs to start working, and older adults with severe depression particularly when accompanied by psychotic delusions. At Duke University Hospital, where I (HK) practice, for example, of the 1,500 ECT treatments done yearly, 70 percent are performed on depressed persons over the age of sixty. Some remarkable recoveries have been seen in older people whom everyone thought were senile and demented and ready to be admitted permanently to a nursing home. After a series of treatments, some of these people brightened up, became functional again, and were able to return home and live independently.

Today ECT is performed with the precision and finesse of a surgical operation. It is extremely safe. During ECT patients typically undergo general anesthesia and muscle paralysis so that they do not physically convulse (the seizure takes place only in the brain). An anesthesiologist and sometimes a cardiologist are present along with the psychiatrist who administers the treatment. A small electrical charge is applied to only one-half of the brain, the nondominant side, to induce a brief seizure. The patient sleeps during the procedure and has no memory of the event. Between eight and twelve treatments over a three-week period are necessary for complete remission of depression. Treatments are so safe now that they are often administered to outpatients without hospitalization.

Following is one patient's account of her struggle with bipolar disorder, including the role of ECT treatments in her return to healthier functioning.

From Torment to Thanksgiving

"The first signs of depression started when I was fourteen years old, shortly after my father was diagnosed with bone cancer, which left him disabled and periodically bed ridden for the next ten years. Our family was devastated. My mother was a wreck, and my only sibling, a sister three years older than me, distanced herself from the situation. My mother and I became the primary caregivers for my father. I regularly emptied urinals and spit-trays and spoon-fed him when he was in too much pain or too weak from the chemo to lift his arms. It was a whole lot of depressing drama and responsibility for a fourteen-year-old.

"When I was fifteen I started drinking alcohol, smoking cigarettes, and then smoking marijuana, which turned out to be my saving grace. Marijuana was like a godsend to me because it made me feel better. It lifted me out of the depression I was struggling with and provided the feeling that even though life was awful, everything would be okay. Marijuana was my antidepressant. Before long I was getting drunk and high every weekend and eventually smoking marijuana daily. Surprisingly, I was still getting good grades in school, cheerleading, working part-time, and helping my mother take care of my father and the house. The drugs and alcohol, although occasionally causing some havoc, were an effective way for me to self-medicate and continue to function and satisfy responsibilities.

"I graduated high school and attended a university about forty-five minutes from home—far enough away to not live at home, but close enough to regularly come home to visit my family and care for my father. My D & A (drug and alcohol) use progressed, and I started experimenting with LSD and cocaine. When I was twenty-two and a senior in college, the D & A use caught up to me. It stopped 'fixing me' as it had before, and I experienced my first major depression. A family doctor put me on Prozac for the depression; however, I continued the D & A use, which caused a psychotic episode with severe paranoia, resulting in my first hospitalization. I was released from the hospital two weeks later, but I continued to use D & A while taking medication. I withdrew from school because my grades were beginning to suffer. I became estranged from my parents, convinced they were part of a satanic cult because of their involvement in the Masonic order.

"In October 1991 I was hospitalized again in a state of psychosis and depression. After several weeks in the hospital I reconciled with my parents (mostly so I could leave the hospital and live with them) on the condition that I admit I had a problem with D & A, stop using, and agree to attend AA (Alcoholics Anonymous) meetings, which I did. My father died three months later. I stayed sober for another four months and then spent the next three years in and out of AA and sobriety, as well as in and out of the psychiatric wards of hospitals. During all this I had a relationship with God and Jesus Christ but regularly fell away and lived in chaos.

"In the summer of 1994 I had been sober for seven months when I decided I did not need my medication any longer. I had been listening to a religious radio station that had a 'Praise in the Night' call-in advice program that aired from midnight to five in the morning. I called in and the minister told me all I needed was God and that I did not need medication, which was exactly what I wanted to hear. I went off the meds and became even more manic, ending up in Florida. After several months I got sober again, regained my sanity, fell into a severe depression, and begged my mother to allow me to return home, which she did.

"I was hospitalized for the last time in January 1995 after I had been sober for six months. Hope became a major factor for me during this final hospitalization, when I fell into the deepest pit of depression I had experienced. I had been in the psych ward for over two months, cycled on several types of antidepressants to no avail, and did not feel any less depressed than I did on the day of admission. While doing her rounds, one of the young nurses could see the hopeless state I was in. She said: 'I know you feel totally hopeless right now and that things will never get better. But I want you to know that I, too, went through a severe depression. I was so bad I ended up in Central State Hospital (you had to be really bad to go to Central). But I did get better. I was able to go to school and get my nursing degree, and I am doing really well now. If I could be that sick and recover, so can you.' For the first time I actually had a glimmer of hope that I could come out of the pit of hell called depression.

"Another turning point was while I was still in the hospital and my doctor talked to me about God and quoted Romans 8:31, 'If God is for us, who can be against us?' Up to this time, I had a more difficult time accepting the fact that I needed medication and must faithfully follow my doctor's instructions than I had accepting that I was an addict and could never again use drugs or alcohol. This doctor's profession of faith triggered something within me that allowed me to completely trust him and his judgment, which made me an obedient patient, following all his directives and recommendations. He suggested that ECT might help me.

"Since none of the antidepressants were working, I agreed to a series of ECT treatments, which I now know saved my life. I began attending AA meetings again, even before I was released from the hospital. I also began attending daily church services that were held at the hospital and started reading the Bible regularly, praying, and developing my relationship with God. Through it all, I always clung to my relationship with Jesus Christ, and I know that it was because I gave my will and my life to him that he in turn gave me a new life."

"It has been more than seven years since I was last hospitalized and more than eight since my last manic episode. I have not used alcohol or illicit drugs for over eight years. During the time since my last hospital-ization in 1995, I returned to undergraduate school and completed my bachelor's degree, worked for two years in the communications field, then went to Case Western University and graduated with a master of science degree. I am now successfully living on my own and am work-ing as the program coordinator of the substance abuse program for an agency in the criminal justice field.

"All of the above is truly a miracle of God and beyond my grandest dreams when from 1990 to 1995 I was in and out of psychiatric units of hospitals at least eight times. After the depths of torment and despair I have experienced, it is a divine blessing to no longer be in a manic state of constant unrest or in the depths of depression when I felt utterly worth-less and pathetic, without a bit of hope, constantly wishing to be dead. I now have great joy in the many triumphs God has worked in my life, and am thankful that Jesus Christ literally saved me from my torment."

Side Effects and Resistance to ECT

Despite the incredible success and safety of ECT, many Christians and family members resist this therapy, even in the face of severe, life-threatening depression. We believe that this resistance is due to lack of information about the procedure as it is practiced today. That picture of Jack Nicholson convulsing uncontrollably is an image that is difficult to get out of one's mind. The movie industry in general has been largely responsible for the negative public image of ECT. After a review of twenty-two films released between 1948 and 2000, beginning with *The Snake Pit* and ending with *Requiem for a Dream,* investigators concluded that ECT is being displayed more and more as a negative and cruel treat-ment, leaving the impression of a brutal, harmful, and abusive proce-dure that has no therapeutic benefit.[5] Once depressed persons and their families realize how safe and technologically advanced ECT actually is, this resistance usually quickly dissipates.

Nevertheless, there remain valid concerns about this therapy and its side effects. There is concern about memory loss following the proce-dure. For younger persons, memory loss is rare and almost always tem-porary, although spotty memory loss may persist for events that occur around the time that ECT is administered. With advancing age, mem-ory problems and mild confusion may persist between treatments and for some time afterward. There is evidence that ECT may induce loss of memory for some events occurring up to several months before and extending to several weeks after ECT has been completed. Consequently,

There is no credible evidence that ECT causes damage to the brain and no evidence that ECT has any long-term effect on the capacity to learn or retain new information.

people fear that such memory loss may be long-term and permanent.[6] However, this concern has not been supported by careful study of memory changes following ECT.

There is no credible evidence that ECT causes damage to the brain[7] and no evidence that ECT has any long-term effect on the capacity to learn or retain new information.[8] Furthermore, depression itself is associated with memory disturbance and difficulty concentrating, and as depression lifts in response to ECT, memory and concentration both improve. ECT can also be administered in a way that minimizes memory loss—such as the use of brief pulse stimulation, one-sided non-dominant hemisphere electrode placement, and individual stimulus.

Changes in heart rate and blood pressure during ECT may cause problems such as heart attack or stroke for older adults with heart disease. Nevertheless, such complications are extremely rare, and with current practices, ECT can now be used safely in patients with advanced heart disease.[9] If a patient has a history of heart disease, a cardiologist will usually be present during ECT. About one in ten people will experience temporary agitation and disorientation following ECT. This goes away after a few hours or can be eliminated immediately with administration of an intravenous benzodiazepine. The problem can usually be avoided entirely by increasing the dose of anesthetic during ECT.

Other Less Conventional Medical Treatments

A number of other medical treatments for depression are more controversial and less commonly used. These include estrogen therapy, repetitive transcranial magnetic stimulation, and psychosurgery.

Estrogen Therapy

Estrogen therapy is currently under study for the treatment of post-partum (after birth) and postmenopausal depression. In a study of sixty-one women with major depression that began within three months following childbirth, estrogen delivered via an estrogen patch produced a significant and rapid reduction in depressive symptoms during the first month of therapy compared to placebo.[10] Another study of twenty-three women with postpartum depression recruited from emergency rooms found that they had low levels of estrogen before beginning estrogen supplementation. After the first week of treatment, estrogen levels rose and depressive symptoms significantly improved over baseline. After two weeks, nineteen of twenty-three women had recovered from their depression.[11] Thus, in postpartum depression, estrogen therapy seems to have benefit.[12]

In perimenopausal (around the time of menopause) depression, the use of estrogen may reduce the somatic symptoms that accompany menopause, improve mood, and thereby relieve some of the causes of depression at this time. Estrogen may also increase serotonin and norepinephrine activity in the brain of postmenopausal women, thereby correcting a chemical imbalance that menopause may induce. Until recently there was little evidence that estrogen alone was an effective treatment for depression in postmenopausal women, since at least four studies had found no improvement in major depression after estrogen therapy.[13] A more recent randomized double-blind, placebo-controlled study using the estrogen patch, however, found that the depression of 68 percent of depressed women receiving the patch was reduced compared to 20 percent of those receiving placebo.[14] Thus, the treatment of perimenopausal depression with estrogen remains controversial but hopeful. Estrogen may increase the risk of endometrial cancer, breast cancer, blood clots, heart attack, and stroke, so caution is necessary and estrogen use should always be supervised by a knowledgeable physician.

In postpartum depression, estrogen therapy seems to have benefit, but there is less evidence for this in postmenopausal or perimenopausal depression.

Repetitive Transcranial Magnetic Stimulation (rTMS)

Within the past few years a new treatment for depression has been receiving increasing attention.[15] Unlike its cousin ECT, rTMS does not require the generation of a seizure to achieve benefits. As a result, it has the advantages of not requiring general anesthesia and not being associated with even temporary memory loss.

In rTMS, an electromagnet is placed on the scalp, generating magnetic field pulses roughly the strength of those emitted by an MRI scan. The magnetic pulses pass through the skull and stimulate the underlying brain tissue.

As with ECT, the mechanism of action is unknown. However, investigators think that rTMS may increase brain glucose metabolism in the areas between brain cell connections and thereby make them more receptive to the effects of serotonin. In any case, stay alert for this new technology as it emerges.

Vagus Nerve Stimulation (VNS)

Another relatively new therapy, vagus nerve stimulation, is also showing some promise for treatment of drug-resistant chronic clinical depression in Europe and Canada, where it is available for this purpose. In the U.S. the FDA approved it in 1997 for treatment of drug-resistant epilepsy, but it has yet to approve it for treatment of chronic clinical depression.

VNS involves the implantation of a generator (about the size of a tape measure) in the upper left area of the chest. Three wires are run from the generator and attached to the nerve in the left side of the neck. The generator is programmed to stimulate the vagus nerve at regular intervals (for example, for thirty seconds every five minutes) and at a frequency determined by the doctor and patient.

A nationwide clinical trial of VNS was conducted in 1999, coordinated by the Department of Psychiatry at Southwestern Medical Center in Dallas, Texas. Although the study was small (thirty patients), some showed marked improvement in their level of depression.[16]

As with all surgical procedures, there are risks and possible complications. The risks include possible surgical injury to the vagus nerve, carotid artery, or internal jugular vein. Complications include coughing, hoarseness, and swallowing difficulties if the vagus nerve is injured. Infection, bleeding, or discomfort may also occur.

Because of these risks and possible complications, we feel that VNS treatment for depression should be reserved for only the most intractable cases, after nonsurgical treatments such as ECT and rTMS have been tried. However, should further studies demonstrate conclusively that the benefits of VNS far outweigh the risks or possible complications, it may receive FDA approval for treatment of depression and become more widely used in the United States than it is today.

Less Common Christian Therapies

Less conventional Christian therapies for depression may be effective in some cases. When these are combined with more traditional treatments, they may reduce the time it takes for the depression to improve. However, they should never be substituted for more proven treatments in cases of major depression, especially when the depression is primarily biological. No scientific studies have evaluated the effectiveness of these therapies, which include fasting, group prayer and laying on of hands, exorcism, and radical forgiveness with visualization and/or role-playing.

Fasting

Some Christians have tried prayer and fasting in order to break a depression. When Jesus' disciples were unable to cast the demon out of the young boy who was suffering greatly, Jesus said, "This kind does not go out except by prayer and fasting" (Matt. 17:21 NASB). In this case, one should note that the persons fasting were those trying to help the afflicted boy, whose affliction was demonic and not identified as depression. Therefore, it would not be good biblical interpretation to pull this concept out of its context and apply it to yourself, if you are depressed, or to a depressed loved one. Sometimes those who are depressed (and/or their loved ones) can become so desperate for help that they are vulnerable to suggestions from others regarding the depression's source as well as its cure.

Fasting can be a means of attaining heightened spiritual awareness and empowerment for overcoming difficulties or fulfilling a difficult task, although no studies have proven its effectiveness for treatment of depression.

The general principle here, which is supported by other Scriptures as well as several thousand years of religious practice by those of a wide variety of religious persuasion, is that fasting can be a means of attaining heightened spiritual awareness and empowerment for overcoming difficulties or fulfilling a difficult task. Fasting includes forgoing, for a period of time, food or other things that one might enjoy. Its benefits are gained through prayer, Scripture reading, and meditation during the fast. The denial of one's desires can prepare the way for a clearer perception of the presence and will of God. Where fasting involves denial of food, the one who is fasting should be careful to take in liquids adequate to sustain and/or cleanse his or her system. At the very least, this means eight to ten glasses of water per day (64 to 80 ounces, about two to two and a half liters). Some recommend juice fasting for anyone taking medication, as the juices help protect the stomach from any harsh medications. In any case, one's physician should be consulted regarding the advisability of and guidelines for fasting, especially if the patient is taking one or more medications. Your doctor can provide information regarding hydration and other issues related to fasting, including a healthful way to break the fast when it is over.

There have been no studies of the effectiveness or safety of this technique in relation to depression. Also, there is concern that if someone is already losing weight because of depression, fasting may make things worse. We recommend fasting only when weight loss is not an issue, while emphasizing that the physical benefits (such as physical cleansing, weight control, or weight loss) of fasting are not primary goals in any case. If you are under medical treatment for depression, this modality should be employed only with the advice and consent of the physician who is supervising your care. If your physician consents, then you should also seek support from your pastor, elders, or spiritual counselor—all of whom should be willing and able to support in some way your endeavor to break the power of your depression via this spiritual means.

Group Prayer and Laying On of Hands

The apostle James wrote: "Is any one of you sick? He should call the elders of the church to pray over him and anoint him with oil in the name of the Lord" (James 5:14). Although this procedure has not been tested scientifically, it appears to have no untoward side effects and may have great benefit. If you wish to employ this method just as described by James, ask the elders of your church to participate. Depending on the church you attend, these leaders may be required to observe certain procedures or rituals in relation to fulfilling your request. In our view, differing observances are more a question of denominational traditions than of biblical command, but the ceremony involved may be helpful to someone of the same tradition.

If you believe in the priesthood of all believers (i.e., that all believers are equal in the eyes of God), then you may gain as much from gathering a group of trusted, mature Christian friends who believe in the power of intercessory prayer and having them anoint you with oil (perfumed olive oil is probably most similar to the kind of oil James had in mind), gently lay hands on you, and pray for you. In some cases, the laying on of hands may occur only once. Since Scripture does not limit this practice, greater effectiveness may be achieved when group prayer and laying on of hands is done once or twice a week or daily if this is possible. Amazing power can result when Christians come together as a group in obedience to Scripture to seek relief of pain for a brother or sister in the faith.

In terms of putting into practice this passage of Scripture, several other things should be considered. Of primary concern is that it is not acceptable to try to use this or any other ritual to try to manipulate God into doing anything, including healing someone, since we should never put the Lord our God to the test (see Luke 4:12). Also, it should be kept in mind that immediately after James mentions anointing with oil, he speaks of confession of sin and forgiveness, including confessing our sins to one another (corporately), that we may be healed (James 5:15–16). This obviously applies to the one who is sick, but it has implications for the others involved as well, specifically that confession of ones sins in the context of a caring Christian community can have a dramatic healing effect on everyone involved. Finally, some have suggested that the passage described by James depicts the union of spiritual and medical treatments—the confession of sins being the spiritual component and the anointing with oil being the application of the best medicine available at the time. If this is an accurate understanding, it surely supports collaboration between the professions with the goal of healing the whole person.

Exorcism

I (HK) have had other psychiatrists tell me about Christian patients of theirs who have apparently benefited from undergoing exorcism. The "demon of depression" was exorcised from them, with at least temporary relief (several months). Christian psychiatrists have examined exorcism for the treatment of schizophrenia and other psychotic disorders, although they do not report good results with these conditions. The response of depression to exorcism has not been studied scientifically. Only those who are spiritually mature and discerning should ever suggest that a person is depressed because he or she is demonized, due to the unnecessary psychic and spiritual pain this may cause the patient if the assertion is untrue, as it usually is. Our advice, should you feel obligated to offer an opinion in a particular case, is to be quick to listen, slow to speak, and constant in prayer for God's wisdom and guidance.

We believe that demons exist today as they did in the days of Jesus. However, we also believe too many well-meaning Christians attribute to Satan and his minions more influence than they may actually have in the lives of believers. Further, we believe that when a person has been bought at a price—the blood of Jesus—making him or her God's possession (see 1 Cor. 6:19–20) and when the Spirit of the living God resides in his or her heart, it is impossible to be at the same time possessed by a demon of depression or anything else.

It is clear, however, that the Evil One surely seeks to render as ineffective as possible the witness of any person he has lost to Christ, in which case depression would be a useful tool. So when believers are afflicted by the "demon whose name is depression,"[17] the best word for this may be *oppression* rather than *possession*. In such cases, exorcism may take a slightly different tack, while the goal remains the same—to deliver the person, through the power of Jesus, from the influence of an evil spirit. In any event, we see no reason why scientific studies could not be conducted to determine if exorcism is an effective and safe remedy for depression.

In the 1970s the Christian Medical Association (then known as the Christian Medical Society) sponsored a symposium on the subject of demon possession, which resulted in a book with the same title, edited

Amazing power can result when Christians come together as a group in obedience to Scripture to seek relief of pain for a brother or sister in the faith.

We believe that too many well-meaning Christians attribute to Satan and his minions more influence than they may actually have in the lives of believers.

by John Warwick Montgomery.[18] Psychiatrist John White contributed several papers to this symposium and book. In his book, *The Masks of Melancholy,* White includes a chapter on "Sin, Disease and the Devil," where he describes eight cases in which he believes there was demonic involvement. He prefaces the chapter with these comments:

> I believe that certain (possibly many) persons diagnosed as suffering from mental disease are in fact demonized [possessed or oppressed]. Yet I confess that I cannot shed my Western mindset without a tremendous struggle which makes it hard for me to be sure whether demons are present on a given occasion. I also confess that I lack faith when faced with my right to invoke the authority of Jesus and that my pride makes me fearful of looking like a fool in front of my colleagues and students. I make my confessions with shame, though I also want to make it clear that I wait on God, frequently requesting the discernment and authority I lack.
>
> A number of things puzzle me. I am humbled to observe that sometimes brand new Christians are used by God to cast out demons that I have failed to cast out. I am also puzzled that I myself have been used to cast them out, only to realize in retrospect that this is what has happened. I am also bewildered that self-proclaimed exorcists who are to my mind complete fools and sometimes knaves are occasionally able to cast out demons by means of the weirdest rituals. Finally, I am uncertain about my right to remove demons from those patients of mine who seem to be possessed by them and who refuse to give me their consent to deal with the real problem.[19]

Whatever your convictions may be about exorcism as a treatment for depression, especially depression that has not responded to other forms of treatment, White's words should be carefully considered before submitting yourself or someone you love to this method. Despite his experience and expertise in the matter, Dr. White humbly waits upon God to clarify issues related to this matter that he as a Christian psychiatrist finds puzzling, even bewildering, while praying that God will provide the discernment and authority he lacks.

The lesson from this is that if someone boldly proclaims that your depression (or the depression of someone you love) is demonic, remember that not many prophets are actually God's spokespersons and that your tendency to believe them may be influenced by your relative desperation in the face of this disorder. On the other hand, if God could use a donkey to deliver a message (see Num. 22:21–35), we are certain that he can use even the most unlikely human representative to accomplish his will.

Radical Forgiveness

In cases in which depression has resulted from severe psychological or physical abuse to oneself or a loved one, lingering bitterness may have locked the affected person into a state of depression. Radical forgiveness is a strategy whereby the therapist uses relaxation, visualization, role-playing, and sometimes hypnosis to take the person back in time to the original event, where the patient and Jesus confront the abuser. Total and complete forgiveness and release of the abuser is the goal of radical forgiveness. In addition, this release usually also liberates the affected person from the prison of his or her own bitterness.

This type of therapy,[20] similar to the theophostic methods mentioned in chapter 8, should be conducted by a trained Christian professional, especially when hypnosis is used. Our perspective is that radical forgiveness can be helpful in some cases and that when it is employed by a trained psychotherapist (most likely a psychiatrist) who is also a mature believer, the same theological, biblical, and spiritual principles—as well as the conclusions—apply as those we presented in our evaluation of theophostic methods.

> *Total and complete forgiveness and release of the abuser is the goal of radical forgiveness.*

Questions for Reflection

1. What did you find most encouraging about Cathy's story of her journey with bipolar disease?

2. If you know someone with bipolar disease, what do you think might be his or her most difficult struggle(s)?

3. What did you find most interesting or helpful about the detailed explanation related to the various drugs that are not antidepressants?

4. In your opinion, should Christians consider electroconvulsive therapy (ECT)? (If you have any experience with this treatment and you care to describe it in a group setting, please do so.)

5. Of the less conventional Christian treatments (fasting, group prayer and laying on of hands, exorcism, and radical forgiveness with visualization and/or role-playing), which would you be willing to undergo and why?

6. Visualization has been severely criticized by some conservative Christians, as explained in chapter 8. Here it appears again in the context of the treatment called radical forgiveness. If you have experienced this method in a counseling setting, how would you describe the result? If you have not experienced this, what is your opinion about whether or not it is a valid method for believers?

7. Two women affected by bipolar disorder, one named and the other anonymous, shared their stories in this chapter. As you think of the pain they experienced and that sometimes still crouches on the doorsteps of their minds, what do you wish you could do for them?

8. If you were involved in research into their condition, what would you be working toward? If you found a pharmaceutical cure, would you want them to use it?

9. What would you say to them if they were sitting next to you at this moment?

10. If you were to pray for them, what would you say?

11. In your journal, write out any or all of your responses to questions 7–10, including the prayer.

Other Medications for Depression besides Antidepressants

Mood Stabilizers and Anticonvulsants	Indications
Older	
Lithium	Bipolar disorder, cyclic depression,
Valproic acid (Depakote—brand name)	or augmentation of antidepressants
Carbamazepine (Tegretol)	
Newer	
Gabapentin (Neurontin)	Same as above
Oxcarbazepine (Trileptal)	
Lamotrigine (Lamictal)	
Topiramate (Topamax)	

Antianxiety Drugs (Benzodiazepines)	
Older	
Chlordiazepoxide (Librium)	Rapid relief of anxiety or panic
Diazepam (Valium)	
Newer	
Klonazepam (Klonopin)	Same as above, except shorter acting and safer
Lorazepam (Ativan)	
Alprazolam (Xanax)	

Antipsychotic Drugs	
Older	
Chlorpromazine (Thorazine)	Treatment of paranoia or psychotic symptoms
Haloperidol (Haldol)	such as hallucinations or delusions
Newer	
Clozapine (Clozaril)	Same as above, but with fewer side effects
Risperidone (Risperdal)	
Olanzapine (Zyprexa)	
Quetiapine (Seroquel)	
Ziprasidone (Geodon)	

PART 3

LIVING WITH
DEPRESSION

CHAPTER 11

Love
The Crucial Role of Family and Friends

Loneliness, withdrawal, and a sense of disconnection from others are common feelings for a depressed person regardless of how warm and supportive relationships may have been before depression changed all that. As Andrew Solomon says in the opening paragraph of his excellent book on the subject, *The Noonday Demon*: "Depression is the flaw in love. To be creatures who love, we must be creatures who can despair at what we lose, and depression is the mechanism of that despair. When it comes, it degrades one's self and ultimately eclipses the capacity to give or receive affection. It is the aloneness within us made manifest, and it destroys not only connection to others but also the ability to be peacefully alone with oneself. Love, though it is no prophylactic against depression, is what cushions the mind and protects it from itself. Medications and psychotherapy can renew that protection, making it easier to love and be loved, and that is why they work."[1]

No one struggles with the "noonday demon" alone, since all of us exist within a network of relationships, one way or another—from spouse (if married) to extended family to friends to associates at work or school. Whatever relationships a depressed person may have, they are *always* affected by depression one way or another. A spouse may feel guilty, rejected, discouraged, frustrated, or angry. Family members may feel embarrassed, even ashamed. Friends may feel manipulated, confused, or alienated. Associates at work or school may wish to help but feel immobilized because they do not know what to do or say. Everyone within the relationship circle of a person with depression is at risk of being sucked into his or her own black hole of hopelessness, even despair, if they so identify with the depressed person's anguish that it becomes their own.

On the other hand, true healing from depression can only occur within the context of supportive relationships. For everyone who is

A depressed person's relationships are always affected by depression, one way or another.

depressed needs at least one ally, preferably more, who will say in words and action: "I love you, and there's nothing you could do or say that would change that. I am with you now, and I'll be with you as long as you need me. I believe in you. I know that your depression has placed a great chasm between the person you really are and the person you feel you are. But I will try to help you bridge that gap with love—mine and God's—for he loves you and believes in you too. We three are in this together—you, me, and God. And when this is over, together we'll find a way to use the pain to help others."

Love—unconditional love—is the ultimate long-term antidote for depression, for at its core love is connected with faith and hope. Faith is connected with God; hope is connected with God's story, of which our own personal stories are mere sentences or perhaps paragraphs. Knowing that our stories are at least sentences in the divine narrative means that each of us has a contribution to make. The apostle Paul wrote, "Love is patient, love is kind. It does not envy, it does not boast, it is not proud. It is not rude, it is not self-seeking, it is not easily angered, it keeps no record of wrongs. Love does not delight in evil but rejoices with the truth. It always protects, always trusts, always hopes, always perseveres. Love never fails" (1 Cor. 13:4–8).

This chapter will discuss how loved ones can help—sometimes confronting, yet always supporting; sometimes perplexed, but not in despair; sometimes grieving, yet not as those who are without hope. The bottom-line good news is that loved ones *can* help. The even better news for believers is that when they embrace by faith the opportunity to help, they are emulating Jesus, who the Scriptures say would not break a bruised reed, nor snuff out a smoldering wick (see Matt. 12:20)—phrases that certainly describe a depressed person's emotional state. Though the journey with depression may be long, burdensome, infuriating, thankless, and even sometimes dangerous, when we try to help a "bruised reed" or a "smoldering wick" in Jesus' name, we can be confident that he is with us, for *Immanuel* ("God with us") is one of his names.

Ambushed by Love—One Doctor's Story

The developmental aspect of psychiatrist Dr. Stephen Mory's story was included in chapter 1. In terms of his recovery, here is how his family and friends helped.

"I was married to Lorraine in my third year of medical school, and that prevented any depression for the next two years. But in my first year of family practice residency I started getting depressed again during a particularly grueling rotation with a lot of night call that I had not been expecting. I did not identify it as a major depression in 1976, as I was a young doctor, happily married, and a committed Christian, so it was unthinkable to me that I could suffer a clinical depression. I was planning to be the doctor, not the patient.

"I would come home in the late afternoon and just lie on the couch for two or three hours with a pillow over my head to block out any light or sound and any contact with my world, including Lorraine. I was not just a couch potato—I was a couch stone. After about six months of this process, I was looking alive for my workday but dead at home, and Lorraine couldn't take it any more. She stormed into the living room one day, flipped the pillow from my head and said, 'This has gone on long enough! Either you are going to get help or snap out of this!' Since getting help was unthinkable, I 'snapped out of it'—in other words, I said the right things and did the right things, at least for a while.

"The addition of our three children over the next seven years was such a joy, as was the challenge of starting a family practice with my best friend, Dr. Jim McGeary, that I don't remember much depression for several years. But after about seven years I started getting a more severe and more persistent depression again, and Lorraine told me she was concerned about me. I stubbornly resisted the possibility of depression or the need for treatment. Our practice had built up to a five-doctor group, but my original partner and best friend, Jim, was still with me. Lorraine said, 'Why don't you at least talk to Jim about it?' This was a set-up because she had already talked to Jim, and he had already been observing depression, patiently waiting for my denial and stubbornness to soften. When I talked to him in 1988 he gently but firmly persuaded me that I was depressed and that it was worth a trial of an antidepressant, nortriptyline. I came kicking and screaming into my first treatment, ambushed by the love of my wife and my best friend. I wasn't going to come into treatment on my own power, but God lovingly conspired with my friends to set this trap. And it worked. The dose was gradually adjusted upward, and by the sixth week I was depression-free.

"With Lorraine's support, I completed a residency in psychiatry, after which we returned to Pennsylvania. By 1999 I had been completely free of all depressive symptoms for over a year. The use of a biopsychosocial

Love—unconditional love—is the ultimate long-term antidote for depression, for at its core love is connected with faith and hope.

I came kicking and screaming into my first treatment, ambushed by the love of my wife and my best friend. I wasn't going to come into treatment on my own power, but God lovingly conspired with my friends to set this trap.

model of treatment had brought remission—the right medicines for the *biology* of depression, the right therapies for the *psychology* of depression, with the *social* deficits addressed through marital therapy in the context of the strong support system of our family, church, and a positive professional experience in the hospital in which I was serving as chief of the psychiatry division.

"Yet something was lacking. I hadn't fully experienced *spiritual* healing. Biopsychosocial treatment is great, but biopsychosociospiritual healing is even better. Over several years Lorraine had been praying that I would come alive spiritually again. She did this quietly, without my knowing that she was praying for me to rediscover the joy of my salvation in Jesus and the power of the Holy Spirit working in me. Not only that, but she had a whole group of ladies praying the same thing with her in a Tuesday morning prayer meeting! That was a little embarrassing when I heard about it later.

"In 1998 Lorraine and I traveled to Buffalo, New York, at the urging of Christian psychiatrist, Dr. Leeland Jones, to attend a seminar on theophostic ministry, which really touched my heart. In my case I needed to resolve the lie of inadequacy or helplessness based on some earlier events in my life. When I made the trip back to Buffalo a few times to meet individually with Dr. Jones, we prayed over these memories with their strongholds of negative emotions and imbedded lies. As we say in theophostic ministry, 'Jesus showed up.' His light shone through the darkness, and he released me from the old lies. As John 8:32 says, 'You will know the truth, and the truth will set you free.'

"Lorraine and I both began to experience the joy of the Lord's presence more than ever before. I prayed with her over a few strongholds, and she also found a new freedom and victory over fears and anxiety. In my daily work I found there were many Christians just waiting for more hope, more power for healing, so I started doing spiritual healing in one-hour sessions, as much as my busy schedule would permit. Time after time Jesus showed up in miraculous ways and spoke just the right truth to the hurting ones in my practice. It was no longer me helping my patients, but it was the Master. I was just sitting at his feet in amazement, watching him heal people. Lorraine and I noticed that at the end of a long day, if there had been some healing moments mixed in with my more routine psychiatric work, I came home energized, feeling better at the end of a ten-hour day than I had felt at the beginning. Her prayers for a spiritual reawakening in me had been answered by the Lord's healing touch.

"In summary, every step along the path of recovery the Lord worked through my beloved Lorraine. Either she was loudly insisting I see the need, softly turning away my anger, quietly conspiring to get me in treatment, or silently praying for me with other ladies. What I might have once seen in my stubbornness as a trap, I now see as deliverance from the trap of depression. I landed in that safe place under the wings of the Almighty, the only trustworthy source of peace that passes all understanding, which guards both heart and mind in Christ Jesus (see Phil. 4:7)."

In rejecting love, depressed persons may be trying to test the authenticity of the love that is offered, especially by those closest to them.

Specific Suggestions on How to Help

Be Supportive

All depressed persons need psychological and social support. They need someone who cares and who will accept them despite their social withdrawal, irritability, impatience, and difficulty giving love back. While some people may act depressed to gain sympathy or to manipulate loved ones, most depressed persons are not that way because they want to be or because it serves some kind of purpose. Most depressed people are exhausted and overwhelmed most of the time, experiencing depression as an enormous emotional weight that they would do anything to get rid of. They are like the Christian, the man in *Pilgrim's Progress*, weighed down by their heavy burdens of despair.

Depressed people need to feel the love and acceptance of those around them because they cannot imagine that anyone could love and accept them—especially in their current state. This is one reason why depressed people sometimes reject the care of others—they simply cannot believe that someone honestly cares about them. Alternatively, through such rejection depressed persons may be trying to test the authenticity of the love that is offered, especially by those closest to them.

In their comprehensive and practical book, *When Someone You Love Is Depressed,* psychologists Laura Epstein Rosen and Xavier Francisco Amador include a whole chapter on the subject, "When Your Help Is Turned Away." Depressed people, in their opinion, do not mean by rejecting help that "they do not want their needs met. Rather, you [concerned loved one] must learn how to give them what they need in a way in which they can accept it."[2]

According to Rosen and Amador, depressed people often solicit support indirectly (as opposed to asking for help) through activities that actually repel their potential helpers. For example, while a nondepressed person might ask for support directly, "Would you mind handling the kids' transportation this week?" a depressed person might withdraw, sulk, even pick a fight, "You never help with the kids. It's no wonder I'm exhausted all the time."

Indirect communication also can be frustrating for a depressed person, as he or she does not have the energy to invest in trying to figure out what the other person really wants or means. This "depressive dance"[3] may happen because the depressed person is irritable and wants to test the waters first instead of bringing it up directly. This dynamic hinders communication and hurts relationships.

Rosen and Amador cite researchers' hypotheses about why depressed people so often reject help, even from those who love them. First, a depressed person may perceive an offer of help—for example, help balancing the checkbook—as an indictment that reads, "You are inadequate. You can't handle even the simplest responsibilities." Since he or she is already feeling inadequate, denial takes over—"I don't need your help with that"—and the offer of help is rejected even if it is desperately needed.

A second factor is the tendency of depressed people to see everything negatively. For them, pessimism is the eyeglasses through which they view their world. Perhaps you've heard the story about the optimist and pessimist who went duck hunting. When they bagged their first bird, the optimist's dog stepped out of the boat, walked on top of the water to the duck, picked it up, and brought it back. At this point, the pessimist commented, "Can't swim, can he?"

While depressed people may actually value support offered by family and friends, they find it very difficult to believe that *any* help offered by *anyone* can really make a difference. If the help offered is advice, even excellent advice, the depressed person's response may be that following it would not work, that the person should just leave him or her alone, or perhaps that the advice giver just doesn't understand what the depressed person is going through. The more often this happens, the more frustrated loved ones may become, with the result that they, too, withdraw.

A third possible explanation for why depressed people often reject help from those closest to them is that they believe that, were they to accept the help, the structure of the relationship would change forever, specifically, that his or her role would be diminished. Such an idea is especially threatening to a person who has always been self-sufficient, in control, or responsible for many things.[4]

When help is rejected, family and friends should constantly and persistently express in words and actions their care and love for the depressed person. Part of that support involves compensating for the work or responsibilities that the depressed person is unable to carry out, yet doing so in a way that avoids making the depressed person feel even more guilty or inadequate for his or her lack of ability to function normally. This is not easy for family members, but it is necessary.

For example, the husband of a depressed wife might surprise his spouse by bringing home a take-out meal for dinner from time to time so she doesn't have to cook. He might explain, "We all need a break from time to time, and this seemed like a good time to give you one." Or a husband of a depressed wife might say he'd like to spend some personal time with the kids, so he has arranged for her to go to a movie with her friend. He might take her on a surprise weekend vacation, while arranging to have someone clean the house while they are gone, and frame it all in the context of a gift because he appreciates her.

The wife of a depressed husband might arrange to have work done around the house or yard *so gradually and subtly* that he doesn't notice things are being taken care of. (This requires considerable strategizing.) Or she might give him a gift certificate to a sporting goods store or arrange a golf outing with his friends.

The key idea here is to communicate, both verbally and nonverbally, that you know the person's temporary disability is just a symptom of depression—"It's just your depression talking (acting)." Make it clear that when the depression has been resolved, he or she will be willing, able, and welcome, to resume his or her normal roles and functions.

Try to Understand

It is difficult for someone who has never been depressed to fully understand what the experience of depression is like. However, if you've never been depressed, you can try to put yourself in the other person's shoes and imagine what life must be like for him or her. Ask the depressed person to describe what he or she is feeling or not feeling, and then listen—trying to stand under him or her to help carry the burden and see the world as the depressed person sees it.

Effective listening is not as passive as most people think. It requires truly engaging, heart-to-heart, with the person who is talking—or not talking, as the case may be. Many depressed people find it difficult to put their feelings into words, as to do so requires concentration and articulation as well as emotional energy—which they may lack. Thus

*Effective listening
requires truly engaging,
heart-to-heart, with the
other person.*

silence may be a depressed person's constant companion. This is a problem for many potential helpers because they, being unused to silence, end up filling the inevitable conversation gaps with meaningless chatter, confirming in the mind of the depressed person that the speaker truly does not understand or care to understand.

If you want to help, try to tolerate the silence; even better, embrace it with your depressed friend. God often speaks in a still, small voice, which is all but drowned out by the constant background noise of our day-to-day lives. Hermits and spiritual pilgrims often view silence as a gift; perhaps you can learn to do so as well.

To listen effectively, you will have to stifle your desire to try to fix what you think is broken. Many Christians instinctively try to fix everything, as if they have the goods that the other person needs—ten steps to this, seven steps to that. Sometimes they proceed by asking rhetorical questions, giving the answers, after which they leave feeling self-justified that they have done all they could to help. For example, instead of asking how you are and then actually letting you describe how you are, they ask a question like: "Wouldn't you like to know how to blow those dark clouds away?" Most depressed people would surely answer affirmatively. Having opened the door, the one who posed the question then delivers a message he or she heard somewhere, such as "how to rise above your circumstances through the power of faith." The problem with this approach is that most of the time, while such helpers may believe what they have done is good, in reality they were simply answering *their own* questions. Thus, they spent their time speaking mainly to themselves, like the Pharisees of Jesus' day who prayed "to themselves" in the public square.

If you are going to help your depressed loved one, you must give up your agenda, try to discern where he or she is going, and go there too with your heart set on helping. This is very hard and can be threatening, for what if that loved one should say something unorthodox or blasphemous?

Once upon a time, and not so very long ago, I (DB) said something that some consider unorthodox or even blasphemous. It was right after the doctors at Dartmouth Mary Hitchcock Memorial Hospital said they saw brain damage on my second son's CAT scan like what had taken his brother about eight years earlier. In that moment the pain rose up, towered over me, then crushed me to bits. Losing one son had been hard enough; the prospect of losing another was *impossible* to bear. I broke down and cried like a baby, and through my tears, these words erupted from my wounded soul: "If that's the way it's going to be, then God can just . . ."

I share this lowest moment of my faith-life to show that God is not put off by the cries of a broken heart. For that very night, as I drove home to tell my parents about what the doctors had found, God's Spirit reminded me that he had already gone to hell in the person of Jesus in order to redeem this fallen world, of which illness (including depression) is a part, and to redeem this fallen man, me, who had dared to hurl such an angry protest heavenward.[5] It was as if in that moment he took me into his arms and said, "I know you hurt, my son. And I know your words came from agony that I, too, have felt. I love you, and there is nothing you could do or say to change that. And when this is over, you will strengthen your brothers and sisters as they try to carry their own burdens."

God is not put off by anger when it is the most truthful feeling you can express. Many Bible characters were upset with him, but he didn't strike them with lightning. However, God is put off by falsehood. So your role as a helper is to encourage your depressed friend to face and express the truth as he or she perceives it, even if it seems to lead, for the moment, away from faith. For the implication of truthfulness with God in the face of overwhelming pain is that there is a personal relationship involved, and your struggling friend is trying to sort out the implications of that relationship within the context of suffering—just like Job and many other believers through the ages.

Depressed people must express how they feel in their own words, not someone else's. Yet many are convinced that *no one will let them say what they need to say* or be who they need to be, so they become either more frustrated and angry or more guilty because they are, in effect, not telling the truth (usually because of real or perceived peer pressure).

The truth about depression and its pain, has two parts: The first is that sometimes life is abominable (or worse); the second is that a loving God is in control. We can by faith affirm that both things are true, even if we don't understand, in light of our experience, how it can be so. Most religious helpers want a depressed person to affirm only part two of this paradox of faith. However, to move through and beyond depression, a depressed person must understand both these truths even if those trying to help insist on accepting only the second part.

Let's suppose you really want to help and your depressed friend says, "I'm really angry that God would do (or allow) something like this." Our advice is to stifle your inclination to correct his or her theology at this

God is not put off by anger, but he is put off by falsehood.

point. Instead, if such communication occurs, rejoice—not that your friend is mad at God but that he or she is secure enough in your love to entrust to you such intensely personal feelings. This is heart talk, not head talk, so instead of trying to force logic or orthodoxy into the moment, you might say instead, "You know, I really appreciate the fact that you feel comfortable enough with me to share such intimate feelings. Your words are like a gift to me, which I will treasure and not divulge to others. I do want to understand how you feel—no holds barred. Please tell me more."

Beyond listening to your friend, another part of developing understanding is to learn all you can about depression and how it affects people and their loved ones. One step has been to read this book. In so doing, you have become more educated about the subject than are many Christians. There are other Christian books on the subject of depression, though most do not address the relational fallout of depression. Some of the more helpful books that deal with this aspect of depression approach it from a secular perspective, and they often have a lot to offer, especially practical suggestions and a commitment to speaking about this disorder without feeling the obligation to do any kind of spiritual window dressing.

The book *What to Do When Someone You Love Is Depressed* by Golant and Golant is one such helpful book. It begins, "When someone you love is depressed

> . . . you feel lost, afraid, confused.
> . . . you long for the person who was.
> . . . you don't recognize who he or she has become.
> . . . you feel shut out.
> . . . you feel angry and frustrated.
> . . . you feel drained.
> . . . you are desperate for a way to connect.
> . . . you feel guilty and alone.
> . . . you will do anything to help.

When someone you love is depressed, you may experience a wide range of emotions such as these, and more. You may feel shock. You might wish to . . . deny reality. You could be angry. . . . You might withdraw or feel hopeless and depressed yourself. You might even try negotiating with God or with your loved one: "If only you would try harder. . . . If only you would get up in the morning, I'll be responsive to you."[6]

These and other reactions are common to the friends and family of depressed people, including Christians. You are not alone (nor is your depressed loved one alone) in your struggle with the intimidating disorder called depression. In order for your relationship with your depressed loved one to more than just barely survive, you need to become more aware of not only how depression affects those who have it, but also how it may be affecting you, and what to do about this.

Encourage

This important relational word means to fill with courage or strength of purpose. It suggests the raising of someone's confidence especially by an external agency.[7] In this case, you are that agent. Family members, loved ones, and friends should encourage depressed persons—to get up in the morning, to go out to dinner, to go to a movie, to exercise with them, to do those things that their depression is preventing them from enjoying, and to seek professional help if they are not doing so already. Once depressed people get out and start moving they often feel a lot better. Encouraging, however, is not the same as forcing, manipulating, or cajoling, nor will arguing about it help much. In fact, arguing will probably make matters worse. Here, again, discernment is crucial so that your suggestions are made in the right way at the right time, to ensure the greatest likelihood that they will be accepted.

One way to encourage your depressed friend to get out (and to get help) is to find a good depression support group and invite your loved one to attend it with you. Groups like this are becoming more common and are often sponsored by churches. One of our hopes is that this book will be useful to such groups and their participants.

Although you may encounter some resistance to this suggestion, you might be prepared to say something like this: "I just want you to know that I will do anything to help you through this difficult time. But I need to learn what to say and what not to say, what to do and what not to do, so I can be an encouragement and not hurt you unintentionally. I am even willing to attend this group by myself to learn these things, but it would be much better if you would go too. Then we could discuss the experience and what we both learn from it." (This is just an example. Each person should express this in his or her own words.)

When my wife, Ilona, and I (DB) attended the group I mentioned at the beginning of chapter 9, I was so glad she was willing to go along. Frankly I was scared of walking into that room for the first time—scared of having to reveal my anxieties and inadequacies and to describe my journey with depression, which sometimes feels like failure to me. Experiencing the group together reinforced things that we learned by listening and also by sharing our own thoughts and feelings, hopes and fears. From time to time it also provided topics to discuss on the way home (or later) that we might not otherwise have brought out into the open. These subjects were easier to talk about in private because they had already been discussed in a group setting.

I learned a lot from that group, and by being there with me, Ilona learned that "being part of a group of people or even having one person with whom you can be open about the state of your emotions—mind and soul—can help immensely in facing the daily struggles of depression. They can even help overpower the demons that haunt one's heart." We guarantee that if you will participate in a support group with your depressed loved one, the fact that you cared enough to attend with him or her will speak volumes, without any words, about your desire to help.

Here are some other suggestions related to encouragement:

1. Offer to go to the doctor's office with the person; this would involve riding with or giving a ride to the depressed person. Either way, you should plan to remain in the waiting room during the doctor visit (unless the depressed person specifically requests that you be present during the consultation).

2. Telephone the person regularly to ask how they are doing. Again, listening, gently seeking to understand, and providing a loving presence are what is needed, not advice or solutions—hard as it may be to not offer these. Knowing you care enough to call will be an encouragement to the depressed person and will help to convince them that others do love them and are there for them, whether or not they can return that love at this time.

3. Find out what the person's favorite movie is and surprise them by getting tickets to the theatre to see it with him or her (or if it's been released on DVD or video, by renting and bringing it over, with popcorn and beverage) for an enjoyable evening as couch potatoes.

4. If you live with a depressed person, you might write short encouraging notes and put them around the house (for example, under the person's plate at dinner time), under his or her pillow, by his or her toothbrush, in his or her lunch box, and so forth. What you do with this suggestion will depend on your personal style and that of the depressed person. Everybody likes to get mail from friends or loved ones, so if you're not comfortable leaving notes around, then buy or (better yet) create greeting cards with

appropriate messages and mail one of them to your depressed loved one from time to time.

Monitor

People who are depressed may need help in taking their medication on time and at the right dose. They may need help in keeping doctors' appointments—both help remembering to go and help getting there. This is the most monitoring that mild to moderately depressed people usually need.

If your loved one is severely depressed, however, they may need observation to ensure that they eat their meals and do not harm themselves (for example, by ingesting large doses of medications by mistake or on purpose). If the medication they take makes them feel sleepy, they will need to be carefully monitored if they are driving or working in an unsafe environment. In any case, care should be taken when allowing severely depressed people to drive, especially if they are taking medications, since their reaction time and concentration may be off.

Following are a few monitoring tips, by no means an exhaustive list.

1. If you cannot be with the depressed loved one in person, phone him or her frequently to check in. Cell phones work best for this purpose, so if you don't have one yet, this one application should make it worthwhile. You must be able and willing to immediately return to them in person if they fail to answer the telephone or give any indication during the conversation that their safety may be at risk.
2. Arrange to have coworkers subtly monitor the depressed person at work, but encourage them to do so without making it obvious to or uncomfortable for the depressed person.
3. Lock up dangerous medications, and dispense them in small quantities to reduce the risk of overdosing.

Our intent in mentioning suicide again is not to unnecessarily alarm anyone but to help you avoid this heartbreaking, all too common, result of depression. As we mentioned earlier, statistics show that about 15 percent of clinically depressed persons will commit suicide. Logic dictates that some of these must be believers. Yet as psychiatrist John White wrote in 1982, this subject is not addressed very frequently in Christian circles. In fact, there seems to be a conspiracy of silence among believers in regard to suicide as well as depression. "I checked every Christian

The only way to exact meaning from an otherwise futile existence is to connect yourself by faith to God.

reference book in my library," White wrote, "including a systematic theology, Bible dictionaries and other likely theological treatises. Not one said a word about suicide." [8] In 1984 the book *Depression: Finding Hope and Meaning in Life's Darkest Shadow,* by Don Baker and Emery Nester, was published.[9] This book, describing Rev. Baker's depression and Dr. Nester's help, contains five pages on suicide. More recently, the book *Suicide: A Christian Response*[10] was published, offering legal, medical, philosophical, theological, biblical, pastoral, and personal reflections on the subject.

Although Christians have not published much on suicide, secular writers have covered it well. For as Albert Camus wrote, "There is but one truly serious philosophical problem, and that is suicide. Judging

Ten Fables and Ten Facts about Suicide

Fable 1: People who talk about suicide do not commit suicide.

Fact 1: 80 percent of those considering suicide do talk about it in one way or another.

Fable 2: Suicide happens without warning.

Fact 2: Suicidal people give many clues of their intentions.

Fable 3: Suicidal people are fully intent on dying.

Fact 3: Most are undecided but are willing to take a gamble that someone will discover their plans and intervene.

Fable 4: Once a person is suicidal, he is suicidal forever.

Fact 4: Suicidal intentions usually are time-limited.

Fable 5: Improvement after suicidal crisis means the risk is over.

Fact 5: Most suicides occur about three months after improvement begins, when a person has enough energy to act out his or her thoughts.

Fable 6: Suicide is more common among the rich.

Fact 6: Suicide occurs in equal proportion throughout society.

Fable 7: Suicide is inherited or runs in families.

Fact 7: Suicide is an individual pattern.

Fable 8: All suicidal patients are mentally ill.

Fact 8: While extremely unhappy and perturbed prior to death by suicide, many who take their own life would not be judged mentally ill.[11]

Fable 9: Deep religious faith makes suicide impossible.

Fact 9: The despair and hopelessness accompanying severe depressive illness can undermine faith.

Fable 10: Caregivers (family or friends) can always prevent suicide.

Fact 10: People intent on suicide may succeed even when friends and family do everything possible to prevent this outcome. When this happens, it is not the caregivers' fault.[12]

whether life is or is not worth living amounts to answering the fundamental question of philosophy."[13] Camus's point echoes the entire message of the book of Ecclesiastes, with the exception of the final chapter in which "the preacher," after clearly describing the futility of human endeavor, finally turns the whole thing on its head by basically saying that the only way to exact meaning from an otherwise futile existence is to connect yourself by faith to God.

Is it possible that your depressed loved one might consider suicide? Yes. In fact, it is *likely* that he or she will *consider* it, even if it is not as likely that he or she will turn the thought into action. So in the face of this likelihood, how are you going to proceed? Frankly, it's hard to know. One of the answers is community, specifically the community of faith. If it is a community in which one may speak truthfully, a depressed person will be allowed to say that life seems futile, meaningless, and absurd. Having said that, he or she can then affirm the other side of the grand paradigm of faith, that only knowing God can give life meaning and hope. We'll return to this crucial theme in our final chapter.

Is it possible for a real Christian to commit suicide? Yes. But he or she would most likely have to be clinically depressed in order to do so, which by definition means that his or her thinking was distorted at the time. Unfortunately, when believers do commit suicide, those who remain too often suffer additional heartache caused by other Christians. One mother whose son had died of a self-inflicted gunshot wound was told by her brother, a Baptist minister, "I can't absolve him; you'll have to accept that he's probably in hell." You can imagine how this response affected that bereaved mother. Our perspective on this is that while this event was tragic beyond words, God is much more merciful and understanding than we can imagine, and ultimately the issue is between the individual and God.

> ### Warning Signs to Watch For
>
> - expressions of helplessness or hopelessness
> - extreme withdrawal from friends, family, and usual activities
> - talking about suicide or ending it all
> - self-destructive or risk-taking behavior
> - giving away favorite possessions
> - sudden changes in behavior or mood
> - increasing use of alcohol or drugs
> - identification with someone who has committed suicide
> - preoccupation with thoughts of death
> - clear plans
> - previous suicide attempts[14]

What can you do? The first thing you should do, if you suspect that your loved one is seriously considering suicide, is discuss the matter with treatment professionals such as the person's physician, psychiatrist, or counselor, and law enforcement professionals as appropriate. Each will have some practical advice about how to handle the situation should it escalate.

Initially, however, it may fall to you to *assess the risk of suicide,* using the above signs as a starting point. From what you know of this person, are the feelings or intentions authentic? Are the methods readily available? As part of your assessment, you might ask: "It sounds to me like you are feeling overwhelmed, almost desperate to end your pain. Have you thought of ways to accomplish this?" Or, "You sound like you feel that everything is hopeless and that ending your own life is the only way out. Are you considering suicide?"

Most people who are not considering suicide will immediately say, "No. I'm not considering that." If, on the other hand, he or she responds by a period of silence or in any way positively, you must press to know the plan, including the method and timing. This will help you stop a preventable tragedy.

Even if he or she admits to suicidal intentions, you can still say, "But I would really miss you. I can't even imagine what life would be like without you. Can we discuss this?" If you respond in this way (versus threatening to call the police or the hospital immediately), your loved one may be relieved to have shared his or her plans and be encouraged to think that life may still be worth living.

If there is some openness to dialogue, you might try to discover what is so dreadful in his or her life that suicide seems the only way out. Then see if you can together come up with a list of five to ten options or alternatives. When you've created this list, ask the person to choose the most constructive option and try it for the next week, after which you may need to go through the same process again. The important issue here is not whether or not a certain option works, but that your loved one is now living in hope instead of despair.

You should also try to establish a "no suicide" contract in which you agree to resist the depression together, and if the person is tempted to commit suicide, he or she will tell you immediately, any time, day or night. If this happens, implement the plan suggested by the professionals with whom you have been in contact. Remember that preventing your loved one's suicide, if he or she is determined to succeed, is not a matter that falls only to you. From the police station to the emergency room there are people trained to intervene in such circumstances. We encourage you, if you conclude that managing the situation is beyond your abilities, to have a number to call immediately. This may seem disloyal to your loved one, but in the end he or she will thank you.

We reiterate, *all talk of suicide must be taken seriously.* If your loved one speaks of it, even tauntingly, you must calmly respond that there are a few things in life that cannot be ignored, even if they are said jokingly. Suicide is at the top of this list because it is one thing that, if successful, cannot be undone. You could say something like the following to your loved one: "So if you really mean what you're saying, we need to talk it through because, as your friend, I am committed to your best interests, and this option certainly is not in your best interest."

Establish Mutually Acceptable Expectations

What should family and loved ones of depressed persons expect of them? The family should be able to expect that the one who is depressed will make every reasonable effort to get better. They should be able to expect the person to go in for evaluation and follow the treatment plan, whether the plan is to take antidepressant medications at a certain dose and frequency or to see a counselor on a regular basis or both. The depressed person may need to be reminded about this, which is okay.

Family members and loved ones should be able to expect that the depressed person will honor their decisions and actions concerning his or her safety. This includes removing from the house any means by which the depressed person could harm himself or herself, locking up medications so they cannot be taken in overdose, contacting the doctor to admit the person to the hospital if this becomes necessary, and even filling out commitment procedures at the magistrate's office to ensure the person's safety if he or she should become a danger to self or others.

It is not reasonable for the depressed person to expect family members and loved ones to sit by and do nothing if the depressed person's safety or well-being is threatened (for example, if he or she is starving himself or herself to death, refusing to take medications, refusing to go to appointments with the psychiatrist or counselor, staying in bed all day, staying home from work or failing to seek a job while the family suffers, or refusing to make any effort to do anything to feel better). This does not mean, however, that family members or loved ones should dominate or control the depressed person's life or make all decisions for him or her. A balance must be achieved that maximizes the depressed person's autonomy and independence while assuring his or her safety and enhancing the chances for the swiftest possible recovery from depression. Finally, family members and loved ones should be able to expect to be honored and respected by the depressed person. Emotional or physical abuse should not be tolerated in either direction.

In order for all these mutual expectations to be understood and honored, they need to be discussed, perhaps with the help of a social worker, counselor, pastor, or any other trusted ally (see below) who is knowledgeable of the circumstances yet wise enough to function as an objective sounding board. Your mutual expectations should include the issues mentioned above and any others that are deemed important enough. This discussion might need to take place over a period of time long enough to allow for dialogue on each point at which there are differences of opinion.

Enlist Allies

Due to the complex dynamics of depression, when you are the primary caregiver it is easy to begin to feel exhausted, rejected, inadequate, helpless, unloved, and unappreciated. Depressed people may not have sufficient energy or emotional reserve to show much appreciation for what others do for them. In order to avoid burnout yourself, you should enlist other sources of support for the depressed person, including another family member or friends. Try to put the depressed person in touch with a fellow sufferer of the same gender who has experienced and emerged from depression.

Keep Yourself Healthy

Family members and loved ones can better cope with the stress of living with a depressed person by developing a regular exercise regime. Exercise will help you expend pent-up energy and give a feeling of refreshment. You can accomplish this at home if you're reluctant to leave your loved one alone.

As much as possible, you should try to maintain your personal routine during your loved one's depression. For example, if you currently participate in a social or athletic activity on a regular basis, you should do everything possible to continue these things, because they will help you relax and be refreshed. They will also help you retain a realistic perspective on life in general and your life in particular. Even a leisurely walk on a regular basis can help. If you share these times with a close friend in whom you can confide, you will be engaging in therapy the way most people received it before the twentieth century, since long before there were psychotherapists, friends often sorted things out during long walks together.

If you are concerned about leaving the depressed person alone because of safety issues, then arrange for a friend or other family member to spend time with him or her while you are away. During these times away from the depressed patient, you should do things that you enjoy (for example, going with a friend to a movie, going out to dinner, or taking a drive to the beach). Or you might consider spending some time in a secluded, refreshing place for rest and prayer—without guilt. Even Jesus, besieged by the needs of others everywhere he went, often took time to refresh and renew his energies, sometimes alone and sometimes with his disciples (see Mark 1:35; 6:31–32; Luke 4:42). The Lord knew that when he returned the crowds would still be there with their urgent needs, but it seems clear that he also knew that in order to minister to the people, he and his followers needed to stay healthy themselves. Surely this same principle applies to us today when we are in a helping situation that can drain our physical, emotional, and spiritual reserves.

Sometimes it is difficult to find and maintain the balance between responsibility toward the depressed person and responsibility toward yourself. One key factor to keep in mind when weighing these needs is that when the depressed person requires such close monitoring for safety's sake that the caregiver's health is jeopardized, then it is time to consider hospitalization. Time away from the depressed person is necessary so that a caregiver can be refreshed and fully able to meet the depressed person's needs when with him or her again. Otherwise, the result may be two depressed people instead of one.

A Special Case: When Your Depressed Love One Is a Teenager

In our instant-fix world, patience is a virtue, as the saying goes. The word *patient* is from the Latin word "to suffer," or to put it another way, patience hurts. The Scriptures describe patience as part of the fruit of the Spirit of God (see Gal. 5:22–23); in other words, it is not a quality that comes naturally to most humans but is expressed when we allow God's Spirit to produce supernatural fruit in our lives.

One of the periods that try the patience of most adults is when their children are adolescents. If their adolescent children are depressed, then what is typically a struggle can seem like a nightmare as everyone tries to sort out what is really going on. Adolescent depression is more common than most people realize, affecting the adolescent's relationships in all directions.

Studies have shown that approximately 1 percent of children and 5 percent of adolescents experience major depression, and the risk after puberty is twice as high in girls as in boys. Without treatment, an episode of major depression in adolescence will last about eight months. Within two years, 40 percent will have another episode of depression; within five years, 72 percent will do so.[15]

Depressed children and adolescents don't always complain of sadness or depressed mood; instead, they may be irritable, complain of being bored, say they are having difficulty enjoying their usual activities, or have academic or behavioral problems at school. When this happens, it is called "acting out" their depression, since they are expressing it in actions rather than in words. It is essential, as in all cases of depression, that medical illness be ruled out as the first step in the evaluation process. Many medical disorders have symptoms that overlap with those of depression. However, if the problem is determined to be psychological (i.e., not caused by a medical illness such as hypothyroidism or hepatitis), then initial treatment consists of four main steps, and parents should ensure that these are all addressed:

1. The depressed adolescent and his or her parents need to be educated about depression, its causes, how long it will last, and the various treatments available. They should also discuss the risk of suicide (2.6 percent of adolescents attempt suicide each year).
2. The adolescent should be evaluated for level of hopelessness with regard to his or her current life situation and the possible treatments available.
3. A "no suicide" contract should be established in which the adolescent agrees to contact a responsible adult and ultimately his or her doctor should the adolescent feel like committing suicide.
4. Firearms, sharp knives, scissors, razors, ropes, twine, dangerous medications, and anything else that might be used to commit suicide should be removed from the adolescent's home.

According to the article "Adolescent Depression" by Drs. David A. Brent and Boris Birmaher, treatment of adolescent depression is similar to that for adult depression in that it consists of antidepressant medication and certain kinds of psychotherapy. Serotonin reuptake inhibitors (SSRIs) are the first treatment of choice in adolescent depression; 20 mg to 60 mg Prozac per day equivalent dose is recommended, which achieves a 60 to 70 percent response rate. Cognitive therapy is the preferred form of psychotherapy, and eight to sixteen sessions over four months is recommended (often together with antidepressant medication). Bear in mind that 20 percent of adolescents with depression end up with bipolar disorder, and 30 percent have psychotic symptoms that warrant additional therapy.[16]

Janelle, who was almost seventeen when she told us her story, doesn't really recall when she first felt depressed. She just remembered being unhappy most of her life. For one thing, her mother has suffered for years from a very painful, extremely rare condition. As a result, for most of the time Janelle was growing up, her mother's time and energies were more or less consumed by her illness. In addition, their family was very active in the only evangelical church in their little town in New Hampshire, and her father was a church leader who set a high standard not only for himself but also for his children.

Janelle remembers that when she was in her first year of high school things just started to get out of control. Besides struggling with all the adjustments to high school life, including trying out for various athletic teams, Janelle also struggled with guilt that she couldn't help her mother. She found a listening ear and the camaraderie she needed, not from kids in the church's youth group but from another group that helped her drown her sadness in alcohol. By the end of her freshman year, she was drinking more and drinking alone.

By the start of her sophomore year, Janelle cared more and more about dulling her pain and less and less about what anyone, including her parents, might think. Her new friends were happy to oblige. The result was that she got caught smoking marijuana and was kicked off the volleyball team. Her parents made it clear that they were very disappointed and they expected her to straighten up and stay away from those kids who were bad influences.

By then, however, bad influences were only part of Janelle's increasingly complex problem. She was depressed, without knowing what to call it. "Part of it," she explained, "was that I just didn't really care about consequences. I wasn't looking past the next day because I couldn't see myself living more than another day. I was literally living day by day. There was no 'long term,' so if someone said 'Do this,' or, 'Don't do this or else,' it didn't mean anything to me.

"What really sent me over the edge was that once, after a party, my parents really got upset. They came down really hard on me. I felt like a complete failure, especially compared to my dad who is a successful kind of person, hardworking and all. I just knew I wasn't ever going to amount to anything . . . that my whole life was one big mistake. I felt pretty hopeless."

Over a period of months, the sixteen-year-old began to turn her confusion and frustration on herself by cutting her wrists. Looking back at it, she didn't really want to kill herself in that way. She knew there was something wrong but couldn't give it a name, so her deepening depression continued to hang over her like a dark cloud.

"When I started slitting my wrists," she said, "one of my coaches noticed and asked me about it. I just made something up every time. But finally I told him what was going on, and of course he told my parents, who were absolutely shocked. I had already been to counseling, which didn't help much. The counselor would ask me if I was depressed, but I was in total denial, so I said 'no.' I mean, I didn't want to be a crazy person or anything. But I finally suggested to my parents that I probably needed medication."

Admitting the truth was Janelle's first step toward recovery, but her situation got worse before it got better. Her doctor put her on a low dose of medication—low enough that it didn't really help much, but strong enough to interact with the alcohol she kept drinking, further intensifying her depression. Grounded and threatened with being kicked off the track team, Janelle felt isolated and cut off. Every day she came home from school with nothing to do.

Gradually over time, Janelle developed a plan. It started with an idea: *I'm no good. I'll never amount to anything. I'm a problem to everyone, just taking up space, so I should just do the world a favor and take myself out of here.*

Next, her depressed mind formulated specific steps to take: *Most girls take the easy way out—pills. But I want people to remember me not as a weak person but as a strong person. I'll use a gun.*

Once she had a plan, she wrote a note to her friends and family apologizing for everything, apologizing for being in the way, apologizing for *just being.* So this was her way to make things easier on everyone—to make the world a better place.

"Then when I was calling one of my friends to basically say goodbye, my dad heard me talking. He came downstairs and asked who I was talking to, and then he found the note and the whole thing blew up. It's weird, but when I was on the phone, it was as though I stepped out of myself and saw what I was doing, and I just knew that I needed help. That was really the first time I realized how really messed up I was. Even though I knew I needed help, I didn't want anyone to help me. I wanted to do it myself. Strange as it sounds, that's the way I was thinking.

"Another strange thing," Janelle added, "is that my parents didn't freak out; they were just totally shocked. I don't think they knew what to do. So they didn't do anything for three days, which still frustrates me. Then they took me to my doctor, saying that I needed a medication adjustment. I needed more than that, though, which he could tell by the deep gashes and scars on my arms. So he made arrangements for me to see a therapist in a city about an hour away."

Janelle didn't know that she was about to be admitted to a psychiatric ward. Her parents didn't tell her, most likely because they were afraid she would fight their plan. "At first I was really upset about it," Janelle recalls. "I was confused. I thought they didn't care, that they were just dumping me. But it was probably the best thing for me. They didn't know what to do, but I'm glad they did something. I'd rather have them dump me and feel abandoned than to be dead."

Janelle stayed in that psychiatric ward for one very long week. "I was supposed to be there for three days," she says, "but I was really honest with them, because I didn't want to leave unless I was better. When they asked me if I was suicidal, I would say 'yes.' I wasn't going to lie just to get out. But when I saw kids coming in overnight or for a day or two, I started to think that I would never get out of there."

Overwhelmed with a sense of hopelessness, she removed the small razor from her pencil sharpener and slit her wrists again. "Then they took me more seriously," she recalls, "and the doctor changed my medication and gave me a higher dose, and my perspective started to change. I didn't like being there, but I was scared to leave. At least in there I didn't have to constantly fight myself, because I knew that even if I wanted to kill myself, they wouldn't let me. So in a weird way it took that fear away. Also, being in the group sessions was good for me because I could see that my feelings weren't weird since other people had them too. In fact, some of them were more messed up than me."

Janelle remains under a physician's care and sees a therapist from time to time. She believes that the combination of both is important. "You need to be on the right amount of the right medication," she said, "and you have to find a therapist you really like. The one I see now is the fifth one I've seen in the past year. I couldn't stand the others, because I knew they were just going through the motions. If I don't think that someone cares about what I'm saying, I am not willing to talk to him or her. The one I have now lets me know that she cares about me as a person, not just as another appointment. That has really made a big difference in helping me find my way through a lot of things I used to find confusing."

When we asked Janelle what her parents did that was helpful, she said: "I'm glad they finally did *something,* that they finally took me seriously and realized I need professional help. When I get really depressed

I'm impulsive, and that was interpreted as rebellion. When we had a family session at the hospital, for the first time they saw my depression, as my dad says, 'eyeball to eyeball,' for what it was—not rebellion, but depression."

Some teens (and adults) are not as fortunate as Janelle, and they become lost in the wasteland of their depression because they have no guide to help them find a way out. We asked Janelle what other parents could do for their own kids in a similar situation.

"Well, first of all," Janelle said, "let them know they are loved and respected, even if you're extremely worried about what kind of crazy thing they might do next. They aren't insane, you know; they're just crying out for help. So they need to know that your love for them hasn't changed just because they're depressed.

"A second thing parents could do if their kids are really serious about hurting themselves," she continued, "is admit them to the hospital. It's an extreme decision, and they may hate you for a while. At first I thought my parents hated me to put me in there. But then I realized that if they really hated me, they would have let me do what I wanted to do, and I'd be gone. So gradually I realized I really needed to be in the hospital where I could get help. In the end—maybe after a long time—they'll thank you.

"Also, there is a fine line between correcting a kid and always criticizing what they do. Parents can correct them when they're wrong and punish them and stuff like that, but parents need to choose their battles wisely, because if you're on your kids all the time, they'll eventually get the idea that they do everything wrong.

"One other thing," she added. "Parents should not expect the person to be just fine overnight. Don't get frustrated with them if they fall back a couple of times. Overcoming depression can take a long time. I know that after I was at the hospital I went backward and cut myself twice, but I haven't done it since then. Sometimes it's like two steps forward, one step back."

Four Helping Patterns

Family and friends can help a depressed person in many ways. On the other hand, there are certain things to avoid because they are likely to only make the situation worse. We've identified four patterns of helping employed by believers on a regular basis. These are judging, giving advice, identification, and empathy. Only empathy really helps.

The Judge

All you have to do is turn to the book of Job to find this pattern, which seems to be as old as faith itself. Job had good reason to be depressed, and his friends did the best they could to comfort him. At first they did well, for they sat with him on the ground for seven days and nights without saying a single word (Job 2:13). Yet after Job began to describe his pain, an extended session of verbal jousting occurred between him and his comforters, starting with Eliphaz, who replied: "If someone ventures a word with you, will you be impatient? But who can keep from speaking? Think how you have instructed many, how you have strengthened feeble hands. Your words have supported those who stumbled; you have strengthened faltering knees. But now trouble comes to you, and you are discouraged; it strikes you, and you are dismayed. Should not your piety be your confidence and your blameless ways your hope?" (Job 4:1–6).

Most Christians who have been depressed have heard such words from their friends. When someone has fallen into the pit of depression, the judge comes along, polishes his halo, grabs his Bible, and pronounces: "People fall into pits because they have sinned. But if you will yet repent, perhaps the Lord will rescue you." Obviously this type of self-righteousness (it's actually playing God) will not help any depressed person.

The Advisor

Advice-givers, likewise, keep the hurting person at arm's length by offering instructions for overcoming depression. Common phrases they use are: "You ought to," "You must," "You should," and so forth. They may quote Scriptures about the victorious Christian life. They can dole out pious platitudes *ad nauseum*. Most likely they will say things like: "All things work together for good." "Cheer up." "Look on the sunny side." "You're just feeling sorry for yourself; after all, other people have it worse than you." "Don't worry—be happy." "You're being a poor witness for Christ, dragging other people down with you." Or even, "I know how you feel. Here's what you should do about it."

Perhaps it goes without saying, but we'll say it anyway: You cannot know how (or what) others feel unless they tell you, even if you have experienced something similar, because each person's journey with depression is unique. Though the paths may be parallel and have similarities, they are still not identical. So the most helpful comforters have banished this phrase from their helping vocabulary.

If you are going to help a depressed person, only offer advice when you are sure that he or she is open to it. Even then, only deal with one thing at a time lest the depressed person feel overwhelmed.

The Identifier

Returning to the pit illustration, as we mentioned earlier, everyone in a depressed person's circle of friends needs to be careful not to sympathize so much with him or her that the potential helper is sucked into the pit also. While it is true that sympathetic friends are better than no friends at all, the result will be that *everyone* will drown in the slime pit of depression. As the saying goes, misery loves company, which is one reason that bars are so full. Yet if you're going to help a depressed person, you must avoid falling into this trap. Here are a few questions to help you discern whether or not this is likely to happen (or perhaps already has happened):

- Am I driven to solve my loved one's problems?
- Do I feel absorbed by him or her?
- When he or she talks, am I mad, offended, or bitter about the same things he or she is focused on?
- When he or she blames someone or something for the depression, am I in total agreement?
- Do the things he or she shares remind me of my own woes, which I then freely share with him or her?
- When he or she expresses doubts or fears, do I feel anxiety or fear?

The Empathizer

True compassion involves suffering together with a person—indeed, this is the Latin root of the word itself (*com*="together," *pati*="to suffer"). One definition that seems to capture the deeper meaning of *compassion* is: "Your pain in my heart." It is possible to feel deeply someone else's pain and to hurt with him or her to the point that the other's pain is diminished, while remembering that the pain is his or hers and not your own.

Returning to the pit analogy, the empathizer goes and gets a ladder, puts it into the pit, and climbs down to be with the depressed person until he or she is ready to climb out. The key difference is that the empathizer has a goal in mind—not just to feel the depressed person's pain, but to also act in a sense as a redeemer, willing to pay whatever cost there is in order for the other person to be healed.

Yes, you may spend a lot of time in that pit with the depressed person, but when he or she climbs out, you climb out too. When that happens, you can rejoice that you have been privileged to imitate in a small way your servant-Savior, who "being in very nature God, did not consider equality with God something to be grasped, but made himself nothing, taking the very nature of a servant, being made in human likeness. And being found in appearance as a man, he humbled himself and became obedient to death—even death on a cross!" (Phil. 2:6–8). If you are really going to help your loved one through and beyond depression, the only way is to lay aside your rights, by choice, with the goal of serving that person's best interests until he or she emerges into the light of joy again.

The Importance of Community

You will be most successful in helping your depressed loved one when you are functioning within the context of a larger support system that involves his or her family and friends, including those in the church. We are designed by God to function best within the context of community. For some, this is primarily family and friends. For believers, it includes the support of the church. You should not allow yourself to get into the position of having to carry the weight of the situation and the decision making alone. With this in mind, we offer the following checklist for decision making as it relates to the care of your depressed loved one, from the onset of the disorder to and beyond its resolution.

If you use this checklist as a guide in concert with your larger family, your friends, and spiritual advisors/representatives of your church, you should be able to rest in the peace of Christ when the decision-making process is finished. This peace is promised not to those who always make the "right" decisions but to those who bring their requests by faith to God, acting on the wisdom that only he can provide. In this context, his wisdom is best obtained through a cooperative group process. As the apostle Paul wrote, "Do not be anxious about anything, but in everything, by prayer and petition, with thanksgiving, present your requests to God. And the peace of God, which transcends all understanding, will guard your hearts and minds in Christ Jesus" (Phil. 4:6–7).

Decision-Making Checklist

Gather Information
- [ ] diagnosis (including full medical workup)
- [ ] treatment options (medication, psychotherapy, spiritual therapy, social worker, all)
- [ ] benefits versus risks (including side effects)
- [ ] treatment recommendations of attending physician
- [ ] additional professional consultation(s)
- [ ] prognosis (likely outcome, including timeframe)
- [ ] costs and resources
- [ ] urgency of treatment decision

Consider Factors
- [ ] patient's wishes and expectations
- [ ] wishes and expectations of the family
- [ ] patient's biopsychosocialspiritual status
  - [ ] biological
  - [ ] psychological
  - [ ] sociological
  - [ ] spiritual
- [ ] costs and resources

List Principles Involved
- [ ] biblical/theological perspectives
- [ ] patient's/family's value system
- [ ] values of friends, including church
- [ ] medical standards of care
- [ ] psychotherapist's/counselor's standards of care
- [ ] other:_____

List Acceptable Options
- [ ] acceptable by secular standards
- [ ] acceptable by biblical standards
- [ ] acceptable to patient
- [ ] acceptable to family
- [ ] acceptable to church/spiritual support system

Utilize Resources
- [ ] medical
- [ ] psychological
- [ ] family (emotional/spiritual/economic/personal)
- [ ] spiritual (pastor/elders/church)
- [ ] social services
- [ ] financial
- [ ] friends or other agencies:_____

Make the Decision

Make the treatment decision prayerfully after listing, discussing, and resolving the applicable considerations above and any other issues that may apply. When a consensus is reached, ask:

Is it moral (right or wrong according to the rules you live by)?

Is it ethical (consistent with the principles that guide you)?

Is it legal (allowed by the law governing you)?

Is it biblical (conforming to biblical commands or principles)?

Is it in the patient's best interest?

Is it in the family's best interest?

Is it wise?

Questions for Reflection

1. Which parts of the apostle Paul's description of love (1 Cor. 13:4–8) might be most difficult to practice in relation to a depressed loved one and why?

2. Considering Dr. Mory's personal experience with depression, would you be comfortable referring your depressed loved one to him?

3. What do you think was the key to Dr. Mory's recovery over the long term?
   - ☐ insight gained through counseling
   - ☐ equilibrium gained through medication
   - ☐ support provided by his family and friends
   - ☐ release gained through his spiritual experience
   - ☐ all of the above

4. Of our specific suggestions for helping, prioritize which might most benefit your depressed loved one:
   - _____ be supportive
   - _____ try to understand
   - _____ encourage
   - _____ be patient and proactive
   - _____ monitor medication and other concerns
   - _____ establish mutually acceptable expectations
   - _____ enlist allies
   - _____ keep yourself healthy

5. Of the four styles of helping described, which have you personally experienced? Describe what happened, and your reaction.

   - the judge

   - the advisor

   - the identifier

   - the empathizer

6. Of the four styles of helping described, which styles have you used from time to time? Give specific examples.

- the judge

- the advisor

- the identifier

- the empathizer

7. What mutually acceptable expectations would you want to establish with a loved one who is depressed?

8. How might you use the decision-making checklist at the end of the chapter?

Discerning What Type of Help Is Needed

Since depressed people rarely realize their level of depression, it often falls to the family to discern what type of help their depressed loved one needs. Most depressions fall into one of the four categories below. We have suggested some action points for family and friends for each category.

Stage 1: Mood Swings

The loved one has mood swings that last for a few days or weeks and, while interfering with his or her well-being and joy, do not noticeably interfere with relationships, work, or recreation. The family might:

- Be available to talk but not pressure or force the loved one to open up about what's bothering him or her, providing the atmosphere in which such things can be shared without fear.
- Plan a vacation, even if only over the weekend, without the kids. Sometimes simply a drive to the beach or to the mountains will provide time and opportunity for the loved one to open up and talk about what's bothering him or her.
- Listen but do not offer advice unless it is requested. Even then, the depressed person should be encouraged to talk about what options he or she sees available rather than being given a to-do list.
- Do things to relieve the pressure once the reasons for the mood swings are known. For example, if a wife is feeling depressed over having to constantly care for three children under the age of five, the husband might provide child care so she can have a night out with her friends.

As you try to help, keep in mind that action should not be taken to relieve pressure if the action is opposed by the depressed person. However, in view of the loved one's fragile emotional state, you may sometimes need to conceal your real motives. For example, a husband might cancel a business trip to be with his spouse during a difficult time, but he need not say that he canceled the trip just for the wife's sake, for this might add to her load of guilt or self-reproach.

Stage 2: Mild Depression

The loved one has a mild depression that is starting to interfere with his or her ability to function in relationships or work or to enjoy recreation. Depressive symptoms, while not severe, have been more persistent and longer-lasting than in Stage 1. Do everything indicated in Stage 1 as well as:

- Encourage the loved one to talk with his or her minister, see a Christian counselor, or talk with a trusted friend or mature and spiritually wise family member.
- Speak to his or her minister, trusted friend, or family member directly (if the loved one refuses to go) and encourage that person to approach the depressed loved one. This is a bit risky and may upset the depressed person because you have gone behind his or her back. However, as the situation becomes more desperate, it will be worth it in the end.

- Schedule a medical checkup for the depressed person and alert the physician about your concerns.

Stage 3: Clinical Depression

The loved one has a clinical depression that is clearly interfering with his or her ability to function in relationships, work, or recreation. Loss of interest, sleep or appetite problems, difficulty concentrating, decreased energy, excessive guilt, irritability, or social withdrawal are present in various combinations. Do everything indicated in Stages 1 and 2 as well as:

- If the depression is mild to moderate, encourage (if necessary, pressure) the person to seek help from a mental health professional; this person should have either a master's or doctorate in counseling or psychology.
- If depression is severe (five or more symptoms of depression present for two weeks or more) then encourage (and if necessary, pressure) the person to seek help from either his or her medical doctor or (preferably) a psychiatrist who can prescribe antidepressant medication.

Stage 4: Suicidal Thoughts

If the loved one is having suicidal thoughts, either active or passive, do whatever it takes to ensure his or her safety. Active suicidal thoughts include thinking about how the person might harm himself or herself or expressing a desire to do so. Passive suicidal behavior involves failure to take necessary medication, failure to make efforts to eat or drink adequate fluids, drinking large amounts of alcohol, or reckless driving (especially if drinking alcohol). Do everything indicated in Stages 1–3 as well as:

- Call the medical doctor or psychiatrist who is managing the patient's care.
- Remove anything in the house that may be used in a suicide attempt (large knives, guns, ropes, etc.).
- Place all medication in a locked cabinet and keep the key away from the depressed person.
- If necessary, go to the magistrate's office at the local courthouse and fill out commitment papers.
- If you are convinced that danger is imminent, call 911.

Unfortunately, if a depressed person waits too long to seek professional help, his or her depression may worsen to the point that the person loses his or her ability to make rational decisions. The depressed person may quit his or her job, seek to divorce a spouse, or make unwise business decisions, all because his or her judgment has become clouded by the depression. The culmination of clouded judgment occurs when the depressed person starts feeling there is absolutely no hope of ever feeling better, that he or she is eternally trapped in the situation, and concludes there is no other way out of the pain except to take his or her own life. Strange as it may sound, once this decision has been reached, a person may seem to cheer up or exhibit diminished symptoms of depression.

Do not be deceived. Once depression has worsened to this point, it seems that the person is being drawn slowly towards suicide, as though suicide is actually courting or wooing him or her, tempting the depressed person to take things into his or her own hands and finally end the suffering.

William Styron described one effect of this phenomenon: "In truth many of the artifacts of my house had become potential devices for my own destruction: the attic rafters (and an outside maple or two) a means to hang myself, the garage a place to inhale carbon monoxide, the bathtub a vessel to receive the flow from my opened arteries. The kitchen knives in their drawers had but one purpose for me."[17] If your loved one ever refers to objects in or around your place of residence in this odd way, and you are confident that he or she is serious, you should intervene in some definitive way, or you may regret forever that you did not.

CHAPTER 12

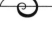

Faith

Acknowledging Depression's Gifts

Internationally known hand surgeon Dr. Paul Brand wrote a book with Philip Yancey, which was originally entitled *Pain: The Gift Nobody Wants*. The title was later changed to *The Gift of Pain*. In it Dr. Brand, who pioneered surgical work with leprosy patients, describes how important physical pain is for our survival because it protects us from injury (or further injury, once we have injured ourselves). People with leprosy lose their ability to sense pain in their extremities. Consequently, they end up repeatedly injuring their feet and hands, to the point where they lose fingers or toes, end up with gross deformity, or sometimes lose a hand or foot. Most of them, given the choice, would wish to recover their ability to experience pain.

Although psychic pain is different from physical pain, is it not possible that psychic pain, including depression, can also serve a good purpose? The answer is "yes," it can serve many good purposes. Depending upon our response to this type of suffering, depression can promote growth in a number of ways that result in positive consequences. For as Peter Kreeft says: "Love somehow goes with suffering. Freedom goes with suffering. Truth, wisdom, and knowledge of reality go with suffering. It seems that everything that has intrinsic value, everything that cannot be bought or negotiated or compromised or relativized or reduced goes with suffering.[1]

In this chapter we describe several good purposes that depression can serve. This list is not exhaustive but a summary based on our own experiences and the experiences of some of our comrades on the *"via dolorosa"* (the way of suffering of Jesus, traced by pilgrims today from the place of his condemnation to the tomb). We do not mean to say that the psychic pain of depression feels good (that would be masochism) or

257

Depression can be a cocoon through which God makes something beautiful out of what is otherwise, for many, very ugly.

that this pain is even good in itself. What we want to affirm is that in the lives of God's children, his grace can transform even the most abject pain into good because he is greater than and his love for us stronger than anything the Evil One sends our way. Satan's objective is our demise—spiritually, emotionally, relationally, and physically. God's primary objective is our growth toward Christlikeness.

The key factor in which direction our depression takes us is our attitude toward it. If we see it as an intrusion and are offended, our pain will increase. If we view it as a gift, not in itself but because of what God can do with it in us and through us, depression can be like a cocoon in which a caterpillar is transformed into a butterfly. In other words, depression can be a coffin or a cocoon through which God makes something beautiful out of what is otherwise, for many, very ugly.

Greater Sensitivity

Depression often occurs in people who are emotionally sensitive—vulnerable to negative events in their lives. They feel deeply hurt when others reject or ignore them or when they fail or experience any kind of insult to their self-esteem. Emotional sensitivity, then, would seem to be nothing but a curse. A broader perspective, however, leads to another conclusion.

For example, where would we be if we lost our emotional sensitivity? Would we have the same concern for the feelings of others? Would we be able to sense as easily when someone else is hurting? Would we be as compassionate if we did not know what it was like to hurt? Answers to these questions and others make it clear that while our emotional sensitivity makes us vulnerable to experiencing depression and sadness, it also enables us to sense pain in others and be motivated to reach out and try to help them.

Imagine a world with no emotionally sensitive people. How could we interact with one another? How could we sense when to comfort or encourage others or when to celebrate with them? Without emotional sensitivity, it would be difficult to interact at the emotional level with people at all. Each person would be entirely focused on how he or she could get ahead at the expense of others. It would truly be survival of the fittest.

Indeed, some people have very little emotional sensitivity and, therefore, hardly ever get depressed. Some of them may be churchgoers, but most of them reside in jails and prisons. Some people were so emotionally hurt or damaged at a young age that they learned to turn off their emotions in order to survive. Consequently, they can't really feel another person's pain, and if they hurt somebody else, they say it's the other person's fault. The worst of them even believe that others deserve to be hurt. People like this go through life neither feeling nor expressing emotion, using others or doing whatever they think will help them obtain what they want without regard to how their actions impact others.

By contrast, depression is often an indicator of the emotional sensitivity that enables us to connect with others in pain on a level unlike one who has never had a similar experience. We can actually sense, sometimes even feel the pain that they are going through, and it often creates in us a desire to help. Caring for someone else, especially someone unrelated to you, is an act of kindness, since *kindness* at a basic level means to treat someone else as one's kind or kindred.

One reason women may be more likely than men to become depressed is that most women are more emotionally sensitive than are most men. This sensitivity may be part of the maternal instinct that enables women to care for children and meet their emotional needs when young. Where would the human race be without mothers who cared? Where would people who suffer be if there were no other human beings sensitive enough to care? Increased sensitivity, not only to our own needs but to the needs of others, is therefore a gift that sometimes develops in us because of, not in spite of, our depression.

Alice, who is now a seminary student, described how her perspective on depression has changed through the years. She wrote: "When my identical twin daughters died at birth, my safe secure world was invaded by fear and grief. Depression became my constant companion as I tried first to simply survive each day and then gradually move on towards actually trying to live in some kind of meaningful way.

"Because I have walked a significant portion of my life's journey with Depression as a companion, I have learned to embrace Depression as a friend instead of fighting it as a foe. I am thankful for my journey through (and with) Depression because I have emerged the better for it. Today I am a woman who is more in tune with my identity, my own unique set of strengths and weaknesses, than I ever was before my journey with Depression. I am also a woman who is now better equipped to journey alongside other burdened believers as they try to integrate/reconcile their painful life circumstances with their belief in God."

When Alice walks alongside burdened believers, she's in good company—the company of Jesus of Nazareth, who announced why he had come by quoting these words from Isaiah: "He has sent me to proclaim freedom for the prisoners and recovery of sight for the blind, to release the oppressed" (Luke 4:18). Why God chooses people for this special calling, we don't know. Yet as we take up and live out that calling to "release the oppressed," we, too, begin to feel release and feel the satisfaction of knowing that we are serving our King exactly as he wants us to.

Change and Growth

Without doubt, depression, with its pain and suffering, changes a person from the inside out. Things that once seemed crucial are suddenly shown to be trivial at best, while other things that perhaps were taken for granted before falling into the pit have far greater importance by the time the depressed person emerges from it.

One of depression's greatest lessons is that it paints our attachments[2] in bold strokes against an otherwise gray background. *Attachments* in the sense used here refers to persons, things, or experiences with whom (or with which) we are connected in an emotionally significant way. Some theories of depression correlate the debilitating power of depression in a given case to the degree of the person's sense of loss when an attachment is broken. For example, depression may follow the loss of a cherished pet, possession, person, or position of influence. On the other hand, depression's *results* can be the fear of loss or related anxieties that to others may seem irrational.

Of this phenomenon, William Styron wrote, "One develops fierce attachments. Ludicrous things—my reading glasses, a handkerchief, a certain writing instrument—became the objects of my demented possessiveness. Each momentary misplacement filled me with a frenzied dismay, each item being the tactile reminder of a world soon to be obliterated."[3] Like many with clinical depression, Styron could feel his world—including his mind—slipping away little by little. The momentary losses of objects he valued were but reminders of this process and of the fact that he was powerless to stop it.

Though many depressed people will not experience frenzied dismay over the loss (temporary or otherwise) of reading glasses, handkerchiefs, or favorite pens, most *will* experience a deep sense of loss of something, more likely *someone,* they cared about or loved. Thus, one of the lessons (or gifts) of depression is that the person affected by it will never again take love for granted, although he or she may struggle mightily with the temptation to become so attached to anything or anyone again, since the pain of detachment is so overwhelming.

Another thing depression can teach is that the searching itself—for truth, meaning, security, reality, whatever—is worth the pain it took to launch us on that search. When things are going well and all is sunny and good, most of us aren't searching for anything except ways to maintain the status quo. Then depression strikes and our world is turned on its head.

In *Where the Roots Reach for Water,* Jeffery Smith describes his own journey with depression, at the end of which his depression has led him back to his sociological and spiritual roots. Here are some salient quotes from the book's last few pages:

> I had conquered nothing, mastered nothing, transcended nothing. I had simply settled into something that had been waiting for me— who knows how long?—and made the descent it seemed to require.
>
> In that descent I had lost all sense of myself; but as that alienation persisted, I'd felt replacing my small self a sustaining kinship with other people alive and long dead. And I'd been given a life unimaginable to that former self: now I was in love, and I was trying to live with faith in something unseen, and I was restored to my family. Perhaps there is no unity without mystery; perhaps I had to become utterly disoriented before I could find and inhabit the landscapes that claimed me, my native places.
>
> This is what melancholia taught me: in some landscapes we see unity more plainly from beneath the earth. . . . In any arid and barren place you must splay the roots broad and deep and let them undertake some saturnine burrowing; you must trust them to trawl through the hardpan and clay that will scarcely nourish them, and find their way to water . . . all this oneness begins in those roots, and those roots take shape from their grasp; and that grasp is the shape of faith, the root tunneling blind through the closed dark earth in its ever uncertain— but still unceasing—reach: for water.[4]

Although Smith's book is almost totally secular, by the end of his journey the author had experienced fundamental changes in his spiritual self. Where once his heart longed for what proved to be emptiness, he had learned that the way to real life was to allow his roots to search until they tapped what Jesus called the well of water springing up into eternal life (John 4:14). It is no wonder that Smith does not lament his melancholia, since it was the vehicle that carried him past what he thought was life toward experiencing another life altogether.

God can use a sensitive Christian to be a rich blessing in the life of one who knows pain and sorrow. . . . Someone has said, "To have suffered much is like knowing many languages. It gives the sufferer access to many more people."
—Billy Graham,
Unto the Hills

Depression will
permanently etch the
words: "I need God"
upon one doorpost of
your heart. On the other
doorpost it will etch,
"I need others."

Creativity

Our experience has been that our depression and all the related emotions, wonderings, and wanderings naturally finds expression in creativity of one type or another. That is not to say that we think we were extraordinarily creative before our struggles or that we are now but that our struggles produced creative energy that demanded expression in some way.

Our observation of our fellow strugglers is that, more often than not, their personal pain erupts in poetry, prose, music, painting, or other forms of creativity either while they are depressed or afterward. Although some never show their creative works to others, perhaps because what is expressed is so private or possibly due to fear of rejection, we encourage all who are depressed to allow any creative drive that exists to express itself, as this can be very therapeutic even if no one else ever knows about it.

In *The Secret Strength of Depression,* Frederich Flach, M.D., writes,

> Depressive episodes . . . can provide the individual with an opportunity to become more of a person, more sensitive, more creative, more effective after the depression has lifted. . . . the majority of creative people, whether the term *creativity* is used in the narrow, artistic sense or in the broader sense of being able to see things in a fresh way and to combine concepts in an original manner, will attest to the fact that they have experienced significant episodes of acute depression from which they have rebounded to reach new levels of creativity.
>
> Why is this so? Why should a period of being depressed and feeling hopeless be a prelude to a heightening in creativity? The answer lies in the nature of creativity itself. To be creative in any sense, a person must be able to relinquish old and fixed assumptions that block a fresh appraisal of a situation. . . .
>
> Acute depression is a necessary vehicle for releasing a person from the bondage of such conditioning and freeing the vital elements of creativity.[5]

Philosopher Søren Kierkegaard explained this dynamic: "A poet is an unhappy being whose heart is torn by secret sufferings but whose lips are so strangely formed that when the sighs and cries escape them, they sound like beautiful music. And men crowd about the poet and say to him: 'Sing for us soon again'; that is as much as to say: 'May new sufferings torment your soul, but may your lips be formed as before; the cries would only frighten us, but the music is delicious.'"[6]

Dependence

"Blest are those who know their need of God," Jesus taught (Matt. 5:3 NEB). Depression has a way of permanently etching the words "I need God" upon one doorpost of your heart. Before depression is finished with you, on the other doorpost will be etched, "I need others."

Our struggle with the forces of emotional pain demonstrates forever our inability to conquer such forces by ourselves. We need help, both human and divine. Depression does away with our pride and self-sufficiency, taking the ground of our self-reliance and self-confidence out from underneath us. Both of us can attest to having learned this lesson the hard way.

Sometimes our cry for help may be as simple as, "Lord . . . help!" God, who is not impressed with long, drawn out prayers anyway, responds by lifting us and carrying us over or through our difficulties. One of the paradoxes of faith is that the only way to really know the power of God is to admit our weakness. The apostle Paul described this in 2 Corinthians 12:7–10: "To keep me from becoming conceited because of these surpassingly great revelations, there was given me a thorn in the flesh, a messenger of Satan, to torment me. Three times I pleaded with the Lord to take it away from me. But he said to me, 'My grace is sufficient for you, for my power is made perfect in weakness.' Therefore I will boast all the more gladly about my weaknesses, so that Christ's power may rest on me. That is why, for Christ's sake, I delight in weaknesses, in insults, in hardships, in persecutions, in difficulties. For when I am weak, then I am strong."

Grace is tailor-made for each individual.

Grace

Many who have written about the hidden benefits of depression have mentioned grace. When a person learns about grace through struggling with depression, the word takes on a far deeper meaning than the acrostic often taught in Sunday school: God's Riches at Christ's Expense. Its meaning is far richer than its most common definition, "unmerited favor." In fact, trying to define *grace* is a lot like trying to define *God* or even *depression.*

Sheila Walsh writes in *Honestly:*

> The word *grace* is now as familiar to me as wind or rain, although, as a reality, it is something that was quite foreign to me until recently.

Grace was never meant to be rationed, something we nibble on to get us through tough times. It is meant to soak us to (and through) the skin and fill us so full that we can hardly catch our breath. My problem was that I had such a tight grasp on my life, there was very little room into which grace could be poured.

Grace gave me the courage to face my biggest fears and the harshest truths about my life because it held on to me and never let go. I felt an overwhelming thankfulness deep in my bones. I knew I could never pay for this awesome gift, but it had my name on it, and it would never be taken away.

The joy that springs out of grace is so different from mere happiness. Happy occasions have always helped me forget about the things that make me sad. But the experience of joy is different, deeper, because it knows the whole story. Grace embraced all that was good and true and all that was bad and faithless about me. Grace is love with its eyes wide open.[7]

Debbie Thurman, author of *From Depression to Wholeness*, wrote in private correspondence:

It is said that God gives grace to us as we need it. We can't store it up, though we can remember its effects on us. Some of us need more than others because of our emotional make-up. Inner strength varies from person to person. God's strength levels the playing field, however. In that, there is hope. God draws us to him most effectively through our pain. Here is where we can best identify with Christ, where we can understand what it means to be crucified with him, but also resurrected to a new life that defeats pain and death. It is a life where we gain a deeper sense of who we are in Christ. Romans 8, where Paul talks about our sin nature and its relationship to hopelessness and death, says it very well: Only through the Spirit of God can we have hope to overcome. In John 16:33, the words of Christ also echo this hope: "In this world you will have trouble. But take heart! I have overcome the world."[8]

Our colleague Dr. Stephen Mory expressed his perspective this way: "Depression is an opportunity for grace unlike any other. I wish no one ever had to experience its peculiar power to devastate body, soul, and spirit. The person who has experienced the blackest depths of depression knows the cold power of death and fear that descends on the one who is still living but seems as though dead. He cries out like Paul, 'What a wretched man I am! Who will rescue me from this body of death?' (Rom. 7:24) The answer is in the next verse, 'Thanks be to God—through Jesus

Christ our Lord.' In other words, 'I have already been rescued.' Depressed people know Christ as their deliverer, and rejoice in his coming more than most Christians because they know that no one else could have rescued them from that overwhelming darkness."

In his symphony of wisdom, *Making Sense out of Suffering*, Peter Kreeft quotes St. Therese of Lisieux, "Everything is grace," to which Kreeft adds, "Suffering is something. Therefore suffering too is grace." When asked if he meant that suffering was good, Kreeft replied, "Suffering is made good by grace. Not all things are good but grace makes them work for good. God uses even evils, which he does not do or will but allows because by his grace and our faith working together (he won't do it without us and we can't do it without him) he brings greater good out of evil."[9]

In other words, to equate something evil with the good that God can bring from it is to confuse cause and effect. Something very difficult may be the occasion for growth, and this is good, but the pivotal truth is that the grace of God is so powerful that he can transform even our suffering into something that advances his kingdom purposes in our pain-filled world. His normal way of achieving this is through his people, who demonstrate his existence and redemptive power through their response to or use of their own suffering.

In the new world to come, "He will wipe every tear from their eyes. There will be no more death or mourning or crying or pain, for the old order of things has passed away" (Rev. 21:4). However, in this old world the old order of things still exists, and it remains our privilege to be his ambassadors, begging others to be reconciled with him and showing through our lives the awesome power of this reconciliation through which everyone who believes can become a new creation in Christ (see 2 Cor. 4:1–6:1), itself an evidence of grace, which we are not to receive in vain.

Modern medicine and Christian counseling are also of grace. In other words, in his grace God has granted both knowledge and insight that can restore the bodies and minds of those who suffer from depression to the point where they are able to comprehend and embrace his way, unhindered by debilitating psychic and spiritual pain, which Satan can use as blinders. Thus medicine and psychotherapy can be tools in the Master's hands, not hindrances to his purposes, as long as it is acknowledged that regaining one's physical and spiritual equilibrium is the first step, not the last, in the journey toward wholeness, peace, and joy that are the longing of every depressed believer.

Deeper, More Authentic Faith

Sometimes people who are depressed become disappointed, even angry with God for allowing adversity and the suffering that can accompany it into their lives. They may even think that as a result of this reaction they have lost their faith or committed a really terrible sin. We believe, however, that this kind of truth telling is something God welcomes and honors and that the freedom to tell him the truth (as we see it anyway) is actually a good sign that a real relationship exists, even if it is a relationship in need of reconciliation. Some have found that this kind of open and honest communication with God has opened the door to knowing him more intimately than was ever possible before.

By contrast, many of those who populate church pews today have a superficial understanding of faith, which they think begins when they walk an aisle in an evangelistic meeting or raise their hand in a service with "every head bowed and every eye closed." Some have made the popular "Prayer of Jabez" their mantra, in which case health, wealth, and influence become their goals. They believe, as Job once believed (and probably taught his friends) that good things happen to good people; bad things to bad people. Beyond the fact that this belief is inconsistent with one of the great mysteries of Scripture—that the wicked prosper and the faithful often face affliction—they don't seem to understand that when Jesus called people, his invitation was, "Follow me . . . all the way to the Cross."

Hebrews 11 is sometimes called the "hall of fame of faith," which is defined in verse one as "being sure of what we hope for and certain of what we do not see." Jabez isn't mentioned, but Abel, Enoch, Noah, Abraham (who tried to fulfill God's promise in his own way, through Hagar, for which the Middle East still pays), Isaac, Jacob (a conniver), Joseph, Moses' parents, Moses, the people of Israel choosing to march through the Red Sea, Rahab (a prostitute), Gideon, Barak, Samson, Jepthah, David (an adulterer), Samuel, and the prophets are all mentioned. "By faith" each person or group acted in some way (despite their weaknesses) because they believed God's promise. Yet they all died (except Enoch and Elijah) without receiving the things promised. "They only saw them and welcomed them from a distance. And they admitted that they were aliens and strangers on earth . . . [because] they were longing for a better country—a heavenly one. Therefore God is not ashamed to be called their God, for he has prepared a city for them" (vv. 13, 16).

A few verses later, after naming more names and citing more miracles, the author of Hebrews says,

> Others were tortured and refused to be released, so that they might gain a better resurrection. Some faced jeers and flogging, while still others were chained and put in prison. They were stoned; they were sawn in two; they were put to death by the sword. They went about in sheepskins and goatskins, destitute, persecuted and mistreated—the world was not worthy of them. They wandered in deserts and mountains, and in caves and holes in the ground. These were all commended for their faith, yet none of them received what had been promised. God had planned something better for us so that only together with us would they be made perfect.

verses 35–40

Those who have real faith are sure of what they hope for—that God will keep his word. They are certain that what we do not see—his very existence and the realm of the eternal—is more real than anything that can be seen with purely human eyes or imagined with the human mind.

The author of Hebrews goes on in the following chapter to exhort New Testament believers to keep walking by faith, with these witnesses in mind, fixing "our eyes on Jesus, the author and perfecter of our faith, who for the joy set before him endured the cross, scorning its shame, and sat down at the right hand of the throne of God" (Heb. 12:2). The "joy" set before Jesus was not the agony of the Cross but the fact that beyond that pain was our redemption. In other words, the suffering of Jesus was a means to an end.

These truths resonate throughout both Old and New Testaments. By faith Job could say on the one hand that he wished he'd never been born (see Job 3), followed by: "Though he slay me, yet will I hope in him." "I know that my Redeemer lives." And "when he has tested me, I will come forth as gold" (Job 13:15; 19:25; 23:10). The fire is affliction, and the refiner's fire is hot. Gold is refined at about 1,200 degrees Celsius. Think of that the next time you sing the worship song, "Refiner's Fire." There's a good chance that many of the people around you raising their hands and swaying to the music have not the slightest idea what they are requesting.

The basic issue of faith is not what denomination we are or if we've prayed a certain prayer or raised our hand in a service. Faith's issue today, as always, is: Are you willing to keep walking with God despite the adversity he may allow you to experience, because you trust that in everything he causes or allows, he is motivated by love and acting with your good in

The Prince of Darkness wants you to believe that your life is a mistake and that there is no home for you. But every time you allow these thoughts to affect you, you set out on the road to self-destruction. So you have to keep unmasking the lie and think, speak, and act according to the truth that you are very, very welcome.
—Henri Nouwen,
The Inner Voice of Love

Faith's question is: Are you willing to keep walking because you trust that in everything God causes or allows, he is motivated by love and acting with your good in mind?

mind? If your answer is "yes" and you actually fulfill it (not perfectly, for no one in faith's hall of fame was perfect), others will notice and demand to know the reason for the hope that is in you (see 1 Peter 3:15).[10]

True evangelism (which means "telling the Good News") is when people who have every reason to be bitter and to turn their backs on faith exhibit trust instead. Cynics may see hypocrisy everywhere, but they cannot deny the reality of authentic faith when they meet it face to face. Exhibiting such faith is both our privilege and our responsibility. The apostle Paul described it in 2 Corinthians 4:17 as the "weight of glory" (KJV).

This passage describes the life of faith from the apostle Paul's perspective and experience, which begins with having our souls enlightened by the "knowledge of the glory of God in the face of Christ" (2 Cor. 4:6). This treasure is entrusted to nondescript (and sometimes even cracked) earthen vessels like us and brings with it a responsibility to live our lives for the sake of others so the grace of God will be spread in an ever-expanding circle of impact, one result of which is that its recipients will give thanks and God will be glorified.

Once we have been entrusted with this experiential, not theoretical, knowledge, the task of the Spirit of the Lord is to transform us as much as possible into the image of our glorified Lord, even though from this side we can only see that as if looking into a mirror (or as a poor reflection of the real thing). The Spirit's primary way of accomplishing this transformation, which involves the death of the old self and the emergence of a new self, is to do whatever is necessary to decrease our attachment to the things of this world so the eyes of our faith can glimpse eternal realities even while we are still locked in time and space.

This ongoing process of inner renewal is accomplished in us primarily through our experience of affliction, which feels heavy (like a weight—remember our definition of *depression*) at the time because it is the weight of glory. Specifically, it is the privilege and responsibility to bear witness to the existence of the eternal realm because others will have to confess that only God could transform and redeem affliction like ours into something good.

Where to from Here?

In summary, depression's hidden benefits can include greater sensitivity, growth and change, creativity, dependence, grace, and deeper, more authentic faith. Depression has a lot of power, arising from the restless energy that it generates. We who struggle with depression have the choice of fighting against it, giving in, or embracing it in order to redirect its energy constructively. Because the burden of depression is so heavy, trying to push it away on our own is seldom very successful. Instead, we're better off trying to find ways to use this force positively.

If you are experiencing or have experienced depression, you have an opportunity that nondepressed people do not have. You can connect with others who are depressed at a heart-to-heart level for the purpose of encouraging them (as they will encourage you) to keep walking through the darkness until you emerge into the light of life again. Here are some suggestions on how to do this:

- Be sure you are receiving the best possible treatments (medical, psychological, spiritual, sociological) for your depression. You are a steward of your whole self, not just your body, your money, and your time. Strive to fully utilize all of the potential means of healing that God has made available.
- Call up a friend who is also experiencing depression and share your presence, your attention, and your kindness with him or her. Listen and let him or her know that you understand, but don't give advice or try to provide solutions for the other person's problems.
- Send a depressed friend a note or card of encouragement, letting the depressed person know that he or she is not alone and that you are thinking about and praying for him or her.
- Pray for others who are in difficult life situations and who may be burdened down by their cares. If you are able, offer to pray *with* them about these situations.
- Read some of the Psalms aloud that express how much God loves you and will fight for you. Examples are: Psalms 32:7; 34:17–19; 40:1–3; 112:7–8; 139:1–18.
- Tap any creative energy connected with your struggle and use it to make something—from poems to potholders. It doesn't matter what you make or how perfect it is; the important thing is for you to see that the energy can actually produce something. Once you're convinced of that, who knows where it may take you?
- Purpose to do something kind for someone else every day, starting today.

There are times when the skies are overcast, when spiritual things seem to have lost their meaning and God himself appears to be far away. This is where we are to do battle, to go on actively, and even aggressively, believing in the goodness and purpose of God; never mind what happens or what we feel.
—J. B. Phillips,
The Price of Success

Depression has a lot of power, arising from the restless energy that it generates.

Unfortunately, instead of directing their energies constructively, many depressed people exhaust themselves trying to make things normal again—by which they mean just the way they were before depression changed everything. We've been down that road far enough ourselves to affirm with absolute certainty that one who is depressed can never again have things just the way they once were. This is because depression changes the depressed person and all the people who comprise his or her network of family and friends. Indeed, depression changes the world itself and not just in the way the person views it. We are all part of an interconnected entity called humanity, so when one person experiences pain or joy, the whole is affected, if only to an infinitesimal degree.

On a personal level, as the saying goes, you can't step in the same river twice because the water keeps moving on—so the most reasonable approach is to expect and embrace a new normal. In a spiritual sense, too, all the energy you expend trying to recapture what once was will be wasted. For God dwells in the eternal present, and he invites us to dwell there with him by embracing the now of our lives. Having resolved things in our past that bind, we walk with him toward a future that we can only vaguely imagine in which we will find fullness of joy forever.

Questions for Reflection

1. Do you think it is legitimate to compare physical and psychic pain? Which do you think is more difficult to endure?

2. Which of the following possible benefits of depression have you experienced?
   - [ ] greater sensitivity
   - [ ] change and growth
   - [ ] creativity
   - [ ] dependence
   - [ ] grace
   - [ ] deeper, more authentic faith

3. Of the benefits that you have experienced, which has been the most significant? Which has been the most surprising?

4. We said that the basic issue of faith is: Are you willing to keep walking with God despite the adversity he may allow you to experience because you trust that in everything he causes or allows, he is motivated by love and acting with your good in mind? Record your reaction to this statement in your journal. Before reading this statement, what did you think was the basic issue of faith? If your perspective is different now, how has your journey with depression changed it?

5. Early in the chapter, Alice described her experience with depression, capitalizing Depression as if it were a person with a name. How did you react to this when you first read it? How do you view it now?

6. How do you feel about God's entrusting the "weight of glory" to you?
   ☐ privileged
   ☐ burdened
   ☐ unhappy
   ☐ threatened
   ☐ worried
   ☐ blessed

7. The beatitude that follows "Blessed are the poor in spirit [those who know their need of God, NEB], for theirs is the kingdom of heaven," is "Blessed are those who mourn, for they will be comforted" (Matt. 5:3–4). What do you think Jesus is trying to say here? How might these beatitudes be connected?

8. If grace really is experienced uniquely, how would you describe your own experience of grace thus far?

9. In childbirth a woman is encouraged to move with the pain rather than fight it. In this way neither she nor the baby is hurt. Through our suffering God wants to give birth to a new person. How can you try to move with the pain instead of fight it?

10. Where do you want to go from here? If toward wholeness and joy again, by embracing the pain and moving with it, perhaps you will find it helpful to pray this prayer or make up one of your own.

Dear God,

I covenant with you today that I will do everything I can to seek the treatment I need to help me overcome my depression—whether that be medicine, counseling, or both. Thank you for the wonderful gifts that you have given to science and medicine to relieve the suffering of humanity, including me.

I also covenant with you today that I will try to use the benefits of my depression to further accomplish your goals here on earth, both for my own benefit and the benefit of others. Give me resolve and strength now to bear this burden courageously as Christ carried the cross for me so that I could have eternal life. Help me to redirect the energy of my depression away from its natural tendency to destroy me and hurt the ones I love and toward making me into the kind of person you created me to be—a real person you can use to release captives and free the oppressed. Help me comfort others with the same comfort you have given me.

Finally, though this is hard to do, I thank you for the gifts that you have given me through depression, including the opportunity to come closer to you and the ability to view my own struggles, which I know you understand, with the eyes of faith.

Amen.

Personal Exercise

Your Timeline of Faith

As a way of visualizing the development of your understanding of and practice of faith, on the timeline below register events significant enough to impact your faith either positively or negatively. (You may need a larger piece of paper on which to create your timeline.) You'll be able to fit more in if you identify events with the words written vertically. Each time you make a mark above or below the line for an event that positively or negatively impacted your faith, write your age at that time on the timeline. Make the vertical lines longer or shorter depending on the degree to which each event influenced you.

Each person's timeline will be unique, though there may be some common elements with the sample timeline below.

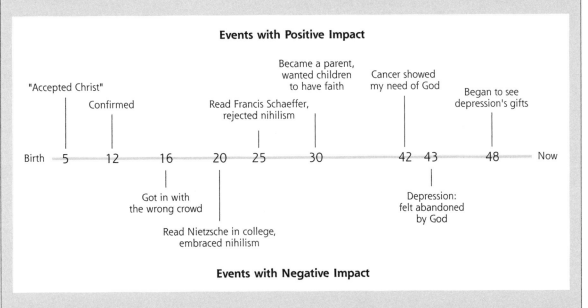

When you're through, connect the end points of the up and down lines, then record in your journal what this simple exercise has revealed to you about your journey of faith thus far.

In a sentence, describe where your faith-journey is headed right now and why.

If your faith-journey is headed in a positive direction, list three things you could do soon to continue in this direction:

1. _____ 2. _____ 3. _____

If it is not headed in a positive direction (or is not as positive as you might wish), list three things you could do soon to go in a more positive direction:

1. _____ 2. _____ 3. _____

CHAPTER 13

Hope
Moving toward Joy Again

Many Christians might be called "smiley face believers." They have never been depressed, and they seem to think that since they are "good people" doing all the "right things," it is God's obligation to ensure they have a nice day. This emotional state is called happiness, which is often confused with joy, which is the fruit of the Holy Spirit (Gal. 5:22–23). If joy is a fruit of the Spirit, it is not a fruit of human endeavor or a result of human experience. Sadly, too many Christians settle for happiness because they don't know the difference, like a person who could have a gourmet meal settling for a greasy burger and some limp fries because it's good enough.

Beyond Happiness toward Joy

When we are experiencing the dark night of the soul—with its arid emptiness and spiritual anxiety—it is nearly impossible to imagine feeling anything other than sadness. Yet when the night is past and the day begins to dawn, many discover that beyond mere happiness is joy, which springs not from circumstances but from the very Spirit of Christ residing in one's soul. For these weary travelers, it is refreshing to learn that the joy of the Lord can be their strength.

Our colleague, psychiatrist Dr. Stephen Mory (whose story has been mentioned several times in this book), described this phenomenon based on his own experience:

"The process of recovering from depression is an opportunity to receive the promised gifts from the Master. He reaches down so deeply in our souls in order to pull out the darkest despair and make room for the good gifts from the Father of Lights, including the joy of the Lord, which now resides at a deeper level than before.

275

True joy rests in the Lord's presence, his promises and his character, not in external events. He is your joy. You are his joy.

"Because the psalmist David had reached the other side of the valley of depression, he could write those familiar words in Psalm 23:4, 'Even though I walk through the valley of the shadow of death, I will fear no evil, for you are with me.' Through his struggles, David had received more courage and assurance of God's comforting presence than he'd ever known before. The Enemy plans that the dark valley will take away everything we have; God allows us to pass through it so he can give us more eternal gifts and promises than we can carry.

"It dawns on a believer while reawakening from depression that true joy rests in the Lord's presence, his promises, and his character rather than in external events. He has promised to never leave. He is your joy. You are his joy.

"No one else can complete the spiritual portion of our healing like Jesus, who trades our sorrows for his joy. These words of Isaiah, fulfilled in Christ, hold the key to this exchange: 'The Spirit of the Sovereign LORD is upon me . . . [to] provide for those who grieve in Zion—to bestow on them a crown of beauty instead of ashes, the oil of gladness instead of mourning, and a garment of praise instead of a spirit of despair' (Isa. 61:1, 3)."

These verses tell where God is going in the lives of his children affected by depression. It is a destination, not a one-night stay; a process, not an event; a journey, the faithfulness of which is determined at any point in time not by how far we've progressed but by which way we're facing—toward God or away from him. If you're affected by depression (personally or through the depression of a loved one), it is crucial to understand and embrace this concept, because while some will be completely cured of depression during their journey, others whose faith is as real and sincere will have to learn to live with this particular "thorn in the flesh" (2 Cor. 12:7).

Yes, there is life and there is joy after depression for some. For others there is joy even *while the struggle continues,* especially as they allow God to transform their pain into power for his purposes as discussed in the prior chapter. For those whose depression becomes a chronic, lifelong companion, there may be weeks or months of remission when joy and happiness seem to be identical once again. However, it would be unrealistic, unhelpful, indeed untruthful for us to suggest that everyone's depression will be cured—even when all available resources (medical, psychological, social, and spiritual) are arrayed against it. In most cases, with proper treatment depression can be managed and living with it can become far better than an endless ordeal. This is why obtaining the best multidisciplinary treatment available and applying it conscientiously is always the most responsible course of action.

Many believers who have never been depressed will disagree with us, and they sometimes express their opinion forcefully and critically to those with chronic depression who are trying to live with it as constructively as possible. The assumption behind criticism of this type may be that the normal Christian life should be one endless ascent up "Sunshine Mountain," when the reality is that for many believers through the ages, the climb heavenward has been made mostly in the dark.

Charles Spurgeon understood this. "We should have thought, judging after the manner of men, that the good were always happy, as one of our children's songs so positively declares," he said.

> [Yet] some of the best of God's people frequently walk in darkness . . . wrapt in a sevenfold gloom at times, and to them neither sun, nor moon, nor stars appear. Some whom I greatly love and esteem, who are, in my judgment, among the very choicest of God's people, nevertheless, travel most of the way to heaven by night. They do not rejoice in the light of God's countenance, though they trust in the shadow of his wings. They are on the way to eternal light, and yet they walk in darkness. Heirs of a measureless estate of bliss, they are now without the small change and spending money of comfort, which would make their present existence delightful. It is idle to attempt to judge a man's real character before God by his present state of feeling. You may be full of mirth, and yet it may be . . . soon over. On the other hand, you may be bowed down with sorrow, and yet it may only be that "light affliction which is but for a moment," which worketh out for you "a far more exceeding and eternal weight of glory."[1]

The life of faith—for those who are depressed and those who aren't—includes both happiness and sadness, successes and failures, joy and pain. What keeps us going is the same thing that kept the heroes of the Bible going—hope. Surely this has been true for us, as expressed in this poem I (DB) wrote after my second son became ill and we thought he might also die:

> I look into the Father's eyes
> And wrestle with a thousand "Whys"
> Why this? Why now? Why him, not I?
> The hurt, the rage, unbridled pain
> Erupting from my soul, again.
> If that's the way it's going to be
> Then build Your Kingdom without me.

Even the darkness will not be dark to you.
—Psalm 139:12

*Some of the choicest
of God's people travel
most of the way
to heaven by night.*

But then, again, where could I go
To hear a word of hope, and know
The promise that beyond the pain
The ballad has a glad refrain
But what for now? And how can one
Still vocalize "Thy will be done"?

And soon I hear a song begin,
Celestial, but from deep within,
A new, yet ancient melody
Of joy *and* pain, disharmony.
Or do the strains combine somehow,
A lovely paradox of sound?[2]

Beyond hope to Hope

In a purely human sense, the word *hope* does not instill much confidence, for example, when you ask if someone is going to be somewhere at a certain time to do something with you and the response is, "I hope so." Your level of assurance that what is hoped for will actually happen is tied entirely to the trustworthiness of the one who makes the promise. In addition, your faith that this or that will happen is also tempered by the knowledge that something unexpected may occur (for either one of you).

Despite its lack of dependability, this type of hope is all that can be offered outside the context of faith. For example, William Styron wrote that

> one need not sound the false or inspirational note to stress the truth that depression is not the soul's annihilation; men and women who have recovered from the disease—and they are countless—bear witness to what is probably its only saving grace: it is conquerable.... For those who have dwelt in depression's dark wood, and known its inexplicable agony, their return from the abyss is not unlike the ascent of the poet [Dante], trudging upward and upward out of hell's black depths and at last emerging into what he saw as "the shining world." There, whoever has been restored to health has almost always been restored to the capacity for serenity and joy, and this may be indemnity enough for having endured the despair beyond despair.[3]

Though we highly respect Styron, and we believe his book is among the best ever written on depression, the wisdom offered has its limits. We've already said that depression's saving grace is not that it can be conquered but that it puts depressed persons of faith in touch with deeper truths about reality, spirituality, and themselves than might otherwise be known. Having one's capacity for serenity and joy restored is little compensation for the agony of despair, much less the "despair beyond despair." The only true compensation for depression has to do with the sense of purpose and fulfillment that comes from redemptive involvement with others in distress, sharing the comfort we've experienced. This is the true route to joy. The rest is mere happiness that will surely evaporate with time.

Viktor Frankl, a Jewish psychiatrist, survived a Nazi concentration camp to write *Man's Search for Meaning,* in which he refers to the perspective the prisoners had to adopt if they wished to survive and help their fellows in despair gain new hope. "I was struggling to find the reason for my sufferings, my slow dying," Frankl wrote. "In a last violent protest against the hopelessness of imminent death, I sensed my spirit piercing through the enveloping gloom. I felt it transcend that hopeless, meaningless world, and from somewhere I heard a victorious 'Yes' in answer to my question of the existence of an ultimate purpose."[4]

Later in the book Frankl adds, "What was really needed was a fundamental change in our attitude toward life. We had to learn ourselves and, furthermore, we had to teach the despairing men, that *it did not really matter what we expected from life, but rather what life expected from us.* We needed to stop asking about the meaning of life, and instead think of ourselves as those who were being questioned by life—daily and hourly. Our answer must consist, not in talk and meditation, but in right action and in right conduct. Life ultimately means taking the responsibility to find the right answers to its problems and to fulfill the tasks which it constantly sets for each individual."[5]

The victorious "yes" heard by Frankl in response to his question about an ultimate purpose comes closer to the biblical understanding of hope, but there is still something missing. For it is one thing to imagine, even become convinced, that there is an ultimate purpose only to link this to the fulfillment of the tasks that life sets for each individual. Clearly life sets no particular task for any individual except to survive as well as possible and then to die. The Scriptures say that life, including all its dreams and endeavors, successes and failures, is empty and futile unless it is centered on God and its hope linked to his promises. In this context, there is a divine "Yes" involved: "For no matter how many promises God has made, they are 'Yes' in Christ. And so through him the 'Amen' is spoken by us to the glory of God" (2 Cor. 1:20).

In a biblical sense, the meaning of *hope* is much different from the best that purely human effort can offer (which is why the second *Hope* in this section heading has a capital *H*). Biblical hope is linked to the promises and trustworthiness of God and to the knowledge that while unexpected (for us) things may happen along the way (such as depression), God is never surprised by anything.

The word *hope* is used over a hundred times in Scripture (up to 186 times, depending on the translation consulted). Its basic meaning is "confident expectation or trust." Here are a few examples, presented in their context to illustrate their relevance to our subject:

> Why do you say, O Jacob, and complain, O Israel, "My way is hidden from the LORD; my cause is disregarded by my God"? Do you not know? Have you not heard? The LORD is the everlasting God, the Creator of the ends of the earth. He will not grow tired or weary, and his understanding no one can fathom. He gives strength to the weary and increases the power of the weak. *Even youths grow tired and weary, and young men stumble and fall; but those who hope in the LORD will renew their strength. They will soar on wings like eagles; they will run and not grow weary, they will walk and not be faint.*
>
> —Isaiah 40:27–31, emphasis added

> I am the man who has seen affliction by the rod of his wrath. He has driven me away and made me walk in darkness rather than light.... He drew his bow and made me the target for his arrows. He pierced my heart with arrows from his quiver. I became the laughingstock of all my people; they mock me in song all day long. He has filled me with bitter herbs and sated me with gall. He has broken my teeth with gravel; he has trampled me in the dust. I have been deprived of peace; I have forgotten what prosperity is. So I say, "My splendor is gone and all that I had hoped from the LORD." *I remember my affliction and my wandering, the bitterness and the gall. I well remember them, and my soul is downcast within me. Yet this I call to mind and therefore I have hope: Because of the LORD's great love we are not consumed, for his compassions never fail. They are new every morning; great is your faithfulness.*
>
> —Lamentations 3:1–2, 12–23, emphasis added

> Therefore, since we have been justified through faith, we have peace with God through our Lord Jesus Christ, through whom we have gained access by faith into this grace in which we now stand. *And we rejoice in the hope of the glory of God. Not only so, but we also rejoice in our sufferings, because we know that suffering produces perseverance; perseverance, character; and character, hope. And hope does not disappoint*

us, because God has poured out his love into our hearts by the Holy Spirit, whom he has given us.

—Romans 5:1–5, emphasis added

I consider that our present sufferings are not worth comparing with the glory that will be revealed in us. The creation waits in eager expectation for the sons of God to be revealed. For the creation was subjected to frustration, not by its own choice, but by the will of the one who subjected it, *in hope that the creation itself will be liberated from its bondage to decay and brought into the glorious freedom of the children of God.* We know that the whole creation has been groaning as in the pains of childbirth right up to the present time. Not only so, but we ourselves, who have the firstfruits of the Spirit, groan inwardly as we wait eagerly for our adoption as sons, the redemption of our bodies. *For in this hope we were saved. But hope that is seen is no hope at all. Who hopes for what he already has? But if we hope for what we do not yet have, we wait for it patiently.*

—Romans 8:18–25, emphasis added

Imagine you were lost and came to a fork in the road with signs that read "Hope" pointing both ways. Beneath the word hope, in fine print one sign says "human," and the other says "heavenly." Which way would you go?

Beyond reality to Reality

We asked some of our fellow pilgrims (most of whom you've already met in this book) to answer two questions: What does joy look like to a believer who has been depressed? How is this perspective different for those who, before their dark night of the soul, thought joy was something else?

We received a number of very thoughtful replies, including the following:

Joy looks like a gift that I didn't know existed or was even a possibility. Joy is something divine and wonderful that makes my days of depression seem a lifetime ago . . . like someone else's life. Joy is the supernatural fruit that was a result of giving my life to Christ!

—Anonymous

The first thing I had to do was to learn to live with it knowing it may be a lifelong illness. But through depression I have learned so much. I had forgotten how much joy could be brought through God's wonders—a baby bird in its nest, the smell of the earth after a spring rain, flowers in bloom, a beautiful rainbow, and snow falling in the winter. These are things I had taken for granted for so long.

At church I no longer take for granted God's Holy Word but seem to soak up each and every word because I know that the next week I may be depressed and down again and unable to attend.

I can finally look at my depression and say that if God has given me this illness so I may help others deal with theirs, it helps to bring joy back to my life and heart.

—Susie

To me joy looks like:

- a rainbow after a great storm;
- a gentle, shining light into a deep darkness (or perhaps the great light that blinds you at first, taking you totally by surprise);
- a ray of sunshine breaking through the dense clouds.
- a tearful smile on a little child's face when he falls off of his bicycle but gets up saying, "I can do this, Mommy";
- being able to stomp in the mud puddles after a terrible storm because you have new wading boots;
- the removal of a pair of sunglasses to discover the glory of your everyday world.

—Alice

I have been able to feel joy even while depressed. I turn on praise music and focus on the attributes and promises of God and allow God to minister to me through the Holy Spirit. Once I understood that depression was not a permanent state for me and one which I can control to some extent by my thoughts, it became easier to take captive my thoughts to Christ. God's Word says that joy is a fruit of the Spirit, and so is longsuffering—longsuffering can be a result of learning to deal with depression. For me, joy is a choice because joy comes through submitting myself to the Holy Spirit: submitting my thoughts, submitting my daily activities, not allowing myself to dwell in depression—feeling depression, but not living in that state. I think having an eternal, rather than temporal, perspective helps us to overcome depression and enables us to experience joy. But most of all, we are to love one another that our joy may be complete. Accepting comfort and love from our sisters and brothers without judgment while we are dealing with depression restores us and helps us "feel" joy.

—Cathy

Jan sent a longer response:

Before my depression I was a person who was always smiling and laughing, mostly happy with my life. If anyone had asked me then what joy was, I would probably have said something like, "Joy in the Lord is being happy all the time because of our salvation. We should even be happy when bad things are happening, since it says in James to count it all joy when you suffer various trials."

Of course, my convictions about this made me feel quite guilty, because when things were difficult I was either sad, depressed, hurt, frustrated, or angry. Then I would think: *But I'm a Christian—Christians shouldn't feel like this.* And in my deepest thoughts, I couldn't quite fathom how to be happy or filled with joy if things were really going bad.

When I went through a deep depression after a friend was killed in a car wreck and then, again, a few years ago, I just couldn't imagine ever feeling good again about anything *ever*. I lost all hope and seemed to be sinking deeper every day. It was like I was enveloped with a huge black fog, and I couldn't possibly find my way out, much less find any hope or care if I even lived anymore. I look back now and realize that even in this state of mind, I really did have hope and joy, just not as most people think of it. My only source of hope and joy then was my longing for heaven and to be with God. I prayed and prayed for God to take me home, but of course he chose not to. Maybe this doesn't sound very joyful or hopeful, but really and truly, a Christian's only real hope is not in this sin-infested world but in the world to come.

Jesus said that this life would be difficult but that he had gone to prepare a better place for us. What better for a Christian to look forward to in hope and joy? In my deep depression, I couldn't grasp that as strongly as I wish I could have, but that still does not negate the hope and joy of knowing heaven will be ours some day. Nor should I have felt guilty (although I did) for not being the smiling, happy Christian I thought I should be.

One mistake I made, I believe, was assuming that joy and happiness are the same thing. Now that I am for the most part depression-free, I can see how my trials have changed my outlook and my attitude. I am not the happy, carefree person I once was. Sure, I have happy moments, and I don't live my life with a scowl on my face all the time, but even if I am not as happy with my life as I wish I could be, there are two things that do fill me with joy and hope: (1) I find joy in being able to reach out to others who have suffered in the same way as I have and to help them in their struggle in some way. (I could never do that as effectively had I not gone through my own struggles.) (2) I find joy in my continued hope for eternal life where all tears and sadness will be gone. I tell my twelve-year-old son, "This life is like a vacation. We get all ready for it and go on the vacation. We have good times and even bad times on the vacation, and then when it's over, we get to go home." Our ultimate hope and joy will be when we finally get "home."

This last point is precisely what drove the heroes of faith on, through the storms and through the night, through terrible persecution, even to death, as Hebrews 11:13–16 explains: "All these people were still living

> *Your capacity for pain is an indicator of your capacity for joy.*
> —David Biebel,
> If God Is So Good,
> Why Do I Hurt So Bad?

by faith when they died. They did not receive the things promised; they only saw them and welcomed them from a distance. And they admitted that they were aliens and strangers on earth. People who say such things show that they are looking for a country of their own. If they had been thinking of the country they had left, they would have had opportunity to return. Instead, they were longing for a better country—a heavenly one. Therefore God is not ashamed to be called their God, for he has prepared a city for them."

Millions of martyrs through the ages have been motivated by this same hope—though this world was not worthy of them, they knew that this world was nothing compared to the one to come. Threatened with torture, death by stoning, hanging, or crucifixion, they turned their back on what they could see and fixed their eyes on what was promised, because they knew God was faithful and would keep his word. Some were burned at the stake, beheaded, burned on crosses, sawn in two, thrown into the fire, or thrown to the lions as the crowd cheered. Why? Because they had hope—hope that this temporal reality is not all there is.

This truth—that we are only aliens and strangers, sojourners on this earth, and that our true home is yet to come—has tremendous power to provide hope not only in our struggle with depression but in every other arena of life if we truly believe it. It is not some "pie in the sky by and by" idea but a central message of the Scriptures. The apostle Peter wrote, "Dear friends, I urge you, as aliens and strangers in the world, to abstain from sinful desires, which war against your soul" (1 Peter 2:11). The apostle Paul uses similar words, "But our citizenship is in heaven. And we eagerly await a Savior from there, the Lord Jesus Christ" (Phil. 3:20).

There is a Reality beyond what we call reality—what we see and experience today. Like hope with a capital *H,* reality with a capital *R* is bigger than temporal reality, which will end, because it is eternal. In an extended comparison of temporal and spiritual realities and their implications for the life of faith, Paul says, "For while we are in this tent [the physical body], we groan and are burdened, because we do not wish to be unclothed but to be clothed with our heavenly dwelling, *so that what is mortal may be swallowed up by life*" (2 Cor. 5:4, emphasis added). Life—eternal life—must be bigger, since it is able to swallow up what is mortal. Three verses later, Paul sums up the perspective involved: "We live by faith, not by sight" (v. 7). This perspective is motivated by hope. As an anonymous author wrote: "Hope is the ability to hear the melody of the future. Faith is the courage to dance to its tune today." In order to dance, one must first hear the music; then one must move one's feet.

Beyond the story to the Storyteller

The book of Job contains one of the most interesting dialogues in the entire Bible. For about thirty-nine chapters, Job and his friends have been arguing about their understanding of faith and God and how he works in our world. The friends are convinced (and try to convince Job) that the greatly distressed and afflicted man must have done something to deserve the calamity that has befallen him. Job maintains his integrity and denies unrighteousness. Yet in the process of what is, at times, a fairly heated discussion, Job has more or less accused God of injustice, since after all, good things happen to good people, bad things happen to bad people, and Job had done nothing to deserve the disaster his life had become.

As you read the story, you can almost imagine God listening in:

> The LORD said to Job: "Will the one who contends with the Almighty correct him? Let him who accuses God answer him!"

> Then Job answered the LORD: "I am unworthy—how can I reply to you? I put my hand over my mouth. I spoke once, but I have no answer—twice, but I will say no more."

> Then the LORD spoke to Job out of the storm: "Brace yourself like a man; I will question you, and you shall answer me. Would you discredit my justice? Would you condemn me to justify yourself? Do you have an arm like God's, and can your voice thunder like his? Then adorn yourself with glory and splendor, and clothe yourself in honor and majesty. Unleash the fury of your wrath, look at every proud man and bring him low, look at every proud man and humble him, crush the wicked where they stand. Bury them all in the dust together; shroud their faces in the grave. Then I myself will admit to you that your own right hand can save you. . . .

> "Can you pull in the leviathan with a fishhook or tie down his tongue with a rope? Can you put a cord through his nose or pierce his jaw with a hook? Will he keep begging you for mercy? Will he speak to you with gentle words? Will he make an agreement with you for you to take him as your slave for life? . . . Can you fill his hide with harpoons or his head with fishing spears? If you lay a hand on him, you will remember the struggle and never do it again! Any hope of subduing him is false; the mere sight of him is overpowering. No one is fierce enough to rouse him. Who then is able to stand against me? Who has a claim against me that I must pay? Everything under heaven belongs to me."

> Then Job replied to the LORD: "I know that you can do all things; no plan of yours can be thwarted. You asked, 'Who is this that obscures

*"My ears had heard
of you but now my eyes
have seen you."*
—Job 42:5

my counsel without knowledge?' Surely I spoke of things I did not understand, things too wonderful for me to know.

"You said, 'Listen now, and I will speak; I will question you, and you shall answer me.' *My ears had heard of you but now my eyes have seen you.* Therefore I despise myself and repent in dust and ashes."

—Job 40:1–19; 41:1–4, 7–11; 42:1–6, emphasis added

Many commentators focus primarily on the last sentence of this quotation from Job. Yet the sentence before it has particular relevance to those who have journeyed a long time with depression (as had Job). Although in God's opinion Job was a model of faithfulness (see Job 1–2), here after struggling so long to understand how things turned out the way they did and especially God's role in it all, Job admits that his knowledge of God before his losses was as if he had only known *about* God. But now he really knows him.

In other words, it was as a result of and not in spite of the sense of loss, anger, and depression that this great man of God became personally acquainted with his Creator. Jesus told a parable of a man who found a treasure hidden in the field. He sold all he had in order to buy that field and possess the treasure (Matt. 13:44). Though Job did not choose to give up nearly all he had—health, wealth, children, even for a while the respect of his wife and friends—in order to know God personally, it happened because he never lost his hope.

Prior to his confrontational dialogue with God, Job had said to his friends, "But I desire to speak to the Almighty and to argue my case with God. You [his friends], however, smear me with lies; you are worthless physicians, all of you! If only you would be altogether silent! For you, that would be wisdom. . . . Your maxims are proverbs of ashes; your defenses are defenses of clay. Keep silent and let me speak; then let come to me what may. Why do I put myself in jeopardy and take my life in my hands? *Though he slay me, yet will I hope in him*" (Job 13:3–5, 12–15, emphasis added).

Millions of our fellow strugglers with depression and other forms of affliction would testify that because they did not lose hope in God and his promises, they were able to keep going step by step—or sometimes inch by inch. This hope did not necessarily allow them to rise above or change their circumstances, but in spite of the darkness, they knew Jesus understood, cared, and would ultimately welcome them into the radiant light of his presence. As your journey-mates and guides, our prayer is that you will have found this hope, for we depressed pilgrims need this more than almost anything else.

The words of the psalmist serve as a fitting benediction from us to you, for they are words that we must often remember ourselves: "As the deer pants for streams of water, so my soul pants for you, O God. My soul thirsts for God, for the living God. When can I go and meet with God? My tears have been my food day and night, while men say to me all day long, 'Where is your God?' These things I remember as I pour out my soul: how I used to go with the multitude, leading the procession to the house of God, with shouts of joy and thanksgiving among the festive throng. Why are you downcast, O my soul? Why so disturbed within me? Put your hope in God, for I will yet praise him, my Savior and my God" (Ps. 42:1–6).

Like the psalmist, perhaps you also thirst for God—the living God—and you used to go with joy to his house. Now you know, as a result of your experience with depression, that the true house of God is the hearts of those who love him. May knowing him and loving him become your source of joy unspeakable and full of glory.

In the memorable words of the poet, Dante, as he returns from the dark depths of hell and sees "the shining world," "And so we came forth, and once again beheld the stars."[6]

Always be prepared to give an answer to everyone who asks you to give the reason for the hope that you have.
—1 Peter 3:15

Questions for Reflection

1. Which promises of God are especially meaningful to you and why? List these, and share aloud if you're meeting with a discussion group.

2. What are the three most important things you have learned through your experience with depression (your own or that of a loved one)?

3. If you agree that there is a difference between happiness and joy, try to define each.

4. What does joy look like to you now? What did it look like before your experience with depression?

5. How are joy and hope connected?

6. What are your favorite verses of Scripture that mention or give you hope? Again, write these down and share them with others.

7. Describe what you think the authors meant by the following: "'Hope is the ability to hear the melody of the future. Faith is the courage to dance to its tune today.' In order to dance, one must first hear the music; then one must move one's feet."

8. After Jacob wrestled with the angel all night, his hip was out of joint. Ever afterward he had to lean upon a staff, which became a symbol of his dependence upon God. Some people think that taking medication for depression is using a crutch. Is there another way to view it?

9. If depression could talk, what would it say to you?

10. If you could talk to depression, what would you say to it?

11. If your experience with depression has been a means of coming to know God more personally, describe the dynamics.

12. Had God given you a choice, beforehand, of finding the treasure hidden in the field in exchange for walking with him through depression, what would you have chosen?

13. What part does trust or hope play in your response?

14. Why is the resurrection of Christ the source of a *living hope* for believers?

15. How is a *living hope* different from other kinds of hope?

16. If you have gained a sense of calling or purpose in relation to depression, describe it in a sentence or two.

17. How do you plan to fulfill this calling? Note: If you feel called to try to help others with depression in some way, write a brief covenant with God about this in your journal. Sign and date it.

18. If studying in a group, share these dreams and pray for one another.

Personal Wholeness Self-Check

Instructions: Complete this survey as you did earlier. Comparing the results may help you visualize changes you have experienced as a result of reading this book.

Wholeness is a dynamic sense of overall well-being—physically, emotionally, spiritually, and relationally—that affects a believer's ability to exhibit qualities consistent with knowing Jesus Christ as Savior and Lord. This definition reflects one of the Bible's key passages describing dynamic faith (see 2 Peter 1:3–11) in which the apostle Peter says that if the qualities of faith, goodness, knowledge, self-control, perseverance, godliness, brotherly kindness, and love are yours in increasing measure, your knowledge of Jesus Christ will be both effective and productive.

Part 1

Estimate your *present* position by giving yourself a score on a scale of 0 to 10 in each area. Respond to the statement for each as best you can. Note: There are no right and wrong responses, only *your* responses. (0 = Not at all true of me; 10 = Very true of me)

1. Mind: I have peace of mind.

   0   1   2   3   4   5   6   7   8   9   10

2. Emotions: I am emotionally healthy.

   0   1   2   3   4   5   6   7   8   9   10

3. Peace with Self: I have a healthy level of self-respect.

   0   1   2   3   4   5   6   7   8   9   10

4. Body: I take care of myself physically, doing what I can to maintain my health.

   0   1   2   3   4   5   6   7   8   9   10

5. Home Relationships: My relationships at home reflect security and love.

   0   1   2   3   4   5   6   7   8   9   10

6. Friendships: My friendships outside my home are mutually beneficial.

   0   1   2   3   4   5   6   7   8   9   10

7. Church: My relationships with people in my church are positive and constructive.

   0   1   2   3   4   5   6   7   8   9   10

8. World: I want my life experiences (positive and negative) to help others in some way.

   0   1   2   3   4   5   6   7   8   9   10

9. Will: My decisions are consistent with my understanding of the will of God.

   0   1   2   3   4   5   6   7   8   9   10

10. Spiritual Maturity: I believe that I am spiritually mature.

    0   1   2   3   4   5   6   7   8   9   10

11. Loving God: My love for God is deep and strong.

    0   1   2   3   4   5   6   7   8   9   10

12. Loved by God: I feel secure (accepted and affirmed) when I think of God's love for me.

    0   1   2   3   4   5   6   7   8   9   10

13. Knowing God: I know God in a personal sense.

    0   1   2   3   4   5   6   7   8   9   10

Your score:

Add your individual scores together. The total can serve as an indicator of your sense of personal wholeness at this time. The divisions below are not based on scientific evidence but on doctoral studies of the tool's author with the help of several friends.

For example, if your total score is:

34 or less: there is room for growth, and we hope that this book has helped you (if so, you might want to read it again or seek assistance in your growth process by other means);

35–64: you may be struggling in some areas, but you are growing;

65–88: your sense of wholeness is probably about average, yet there's still room for growth;

89–117: you feel that you are well adjusted, overall, while also still in process;

118 and up: you haven't left much room for growth, but perhaps as a result of reading this book you have discovered one or two things that could be improved.

Part 2

Using the categories/arenas of life in Part 1, list the three areas in which you think you need the most improvement.

1. _____
2. _____
3. _____

Part 3

To visualize your initial responses in Part 1, record them with an X on the Wheel of Wholeness below. Note: 0 is at the center; 10 at the circumference.

Part 4

Review your responses to the statements in Part 1, placing an O (like a target) on the line under each category to indicate where you would like to be three months from now. Place the O's on the appropriate spokes of the Wheel of Wholeness to indicate your current goals in each area.

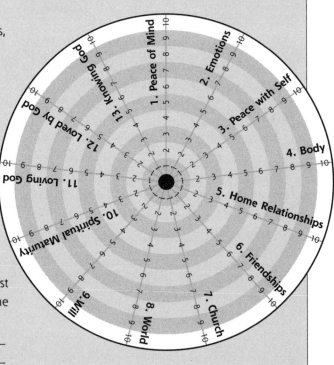

Brief Depression Scale

To evaluate your progress with depression itself, complete the following evaluation again (as in chapter 2) and compare your results.

The following list of statements has been created to help you discern where you are in terms of depression. While it does not try to identify any causes or types of depression, it can be useful to you now, and it may prove useful to you after you have finished reading this book and/or participating in a discussion group that may be studying it.[7]

Directions: For each statement below, circle or underline the response that has described you over the past week.

1.	I often become bored.	Yes	No
2.	I often feel restless and fidgety.	Yes	No
3.	I feel in good spirits.	No	Yes
4.	I have more problems with memory than most.	Yes	No
5.	I can concentrate easily when reading the newspaper.	No	Yes
6.	I prefer to avoid social gatherings.	Yes	No
7.	I often feel downhearted or blue.	Yes	No
8.	I feel happy most of the time.	No	Yes
9.	I often feel helpless.	Yes	No
10.	I often feel worthless and ashamed of myself.	Yes	No
11.	I often wish I were dead.	Yes	No

Scoring:

Count 1 for each response in the first column. Scores of 4 or higher suggest that further evaluation should be pursued with a professional qualified to diagnose and/or treat depression.

Notes

Page 2

1. We are grateful to Roger Norton, upon whose web site this material is based, for allowing us to use it. See: *http://home.att.net/~rjnorton/Lincoln84.html*.

Chapter 1. Like Nailing Jell-O to the Wall

1. Throughout this book, the terms *major depression* and *clinical depression* have identical meaning. The word *clinical* arises from the fact that major depression is usually diagnosed by a trained professional in a clinical setting such as a medical or counseling office.

2. D. A. Regier et al., "The De Facto US Mental and Addictive Disorders Service System: Epidemiologic Catchment Area Prospective 1-year Prevalence Rates of Disorders and Services," *Archives of General Psychiatry* 50 (1993): 85–94; and, R. C. Kessler et al., "Lifetime and 12-month Prevalence of DSM-III-R [*Diagnostic and Statistical Manual of Mental Disorders,* 3d rev, ed.] Psychiatric Disorders in the United States: Results from the National Comorbidity Survey," *Archives of General Psychiatry* 51 (1994): 8–19.

3. M. Olfson et al., "National Trends in the Outpatient Treatment of Depression," *Journal of the American Medical Association* 287 (2002): 203–9.

4. American Psychiatric Association, *Diagnostic and Statistical Manual of Mental Disorders,* 4th ed. [*DSM-IV*] (Washington, D.C.: APA Press, 1994).

5. See, for example, Terrence Real, *I Don't Want to Talk about It* (New York: Simon and Schuster/Fireside, 1998).

6. C. Murray, A. Lopez, *The Global Burden of Disease: A Comprehensive Assessment of Mortality and Disability from Diseases, Injuries, and Risk Factors in 1990 and Projected to 2020,* vol. 1 (Geneva: World Heath Organization, 2000).

7. American Psychiatric Association, *DSM-IV.*

8. See chapter two for more specific details regarding the symptoms of depression.

9. Andrew Solomon, *The Noonday Demon: An Atlas of Depression* (New York: Scribner, 2001).

10. For more details, see David B. Biebel, *Jonathan, You Left Too Soon* (Old Tappan, N.J.: Revell, 1997) and *If God Is So Good, Why Do I Hurt So Bad?* (Grand Rapids: Baker, 1995). Autographed copies are available from the author via e-mail (*dbbv1@aol.com*) or web site (*http://www.hopecentral.us*).

Chapter 2. Depression Is a Whole-Person Disorder

1. Biochemical activity in key areas of the brain can be measured using a Positron Emission Tomography (PET) scan. In this procedure, a positron-producing radioisotope called a "tracer" is either injected into a vein or inhaled as a gas. This tracer—usually carbon, nitrogen, or oxygen—is altered to allow it to emit positrons. The radioactivated tracer travels through the bloodstream to a specific target organ—for example, the heart or brain—where it emits positrons, which collide with negatively charged particles called electrons. This produces gamma rays (similar to X rays), which are detected by the PET scanner and analyzed by a computer to form an image of the metabolism and other functions of the organ in question. A PET scan can show characteristic changes in brain metabolism in those who are severely (and usually chronically) depressed. However, since not all depressed persons have brain changes that are evident via PET scan, the procedure is relatively expensive, and other reliable diagnostic methods exist, PET scans are not ordinarily used to diagnose depression.

2. Chapter 6 provides an overview of types of professional help available.

3. Thomas M. Burton, "Scientists Find Gene Linked to Depression," *Wall Street Journal* (5 February 2003).

4. Caspi, Avshalom, Karen Sugden, Terrie E. Moffitt, Alan Taylor, Ian W. Craig, HonaLee Harrington, Joseph McClay, Jonathan Mill, Judy Martin, Anthony Braithwaite, and Richie Poulton, "Influence of Life Stress on Depression: Moderation by a Polymorphism in the 5-HTT Gene," *Science* 301 (2003): 386–89.

5. The Old Testament book of Job describes Job's struggle with issues like these after losing his wealth, his children, and his health within a short period of time.

6. Henri J. M. Nouwen, *The Inner Voice of Love: A Journey through Anguish to Freedom* (New York: Doubleday/Random House, 1996), xiv–xv.

7. See especially St. John of the Cross, *The Dark Night of the Soul* (New York: Doubleday, 1990).

8. C. H. Spurgeon, *The New Park Street Pulpit* 4: 460, cited by Elizabeth Ruth Skoglund, *Bright Days,*

Dark Nights: With Charles Spurgeon in Triumph over Emotional Pain (Grand Rapids: Baker, 2000), 80–81.

9. Ken I. Pargament, H. G. Koenig, N. Tarakeshwar, and J. Hahn, "Religious Struggle as a Predictor of Mortality among Medically Ill Elderly Patients: A Two-Year Longitudinal Study," *Archives of Internal Medicine* 161 (2001): 1881–85.

10. See chapter 10 for more on this.

11. Lack of sleep, exercise, and a balanced diet leave anyone at risk for health problems including, for some, depression. There are myriad theories and programs promulgated via the internet and elsewhere that promise miraculous recovery from all manner of diseases through the use of dietary supplements. Yet none of these have been scientifically proven to be effective in the treatment of depression, and certainly none is as effective as a combination of counseling and antidepressants, all other things being equal. For those with chronic illness or who have experienced significant weight loss, a good daily multivitamin is probably wise. The only vitamin deficiency that is linked with depression is B-12 deficiency, which is particularly common among older adults who may have difficulty absorbing this vitamin from food. Typically, B-12 is replaced by monthly injections because a multivitamin or even B-vitamin pill once daily will not be sufficient.

12. *DSM-IV* is the abbreviation for *Diagnostic and Statistical Manual of Mental Disorders,* 4th ed. (Washington, D.C.: American Psychiatric Association Press, 1994).

13. See *http://www.cfsan.fda.gov/~lrd/fr990708.html.*

14. See *http://www.cfsan.fda.gov/~lrd/fr990708.html.*

15. From the WHO web site: *http://www.who.int/en/,* "Preamble to the Constitution of the World Health Organization as adopted by the International Health Conference, New York, 19–22 June, 1946; signed on 22 July 1946 by the representatives of 61 States (Official Records of the World Health Organization, no. 2, p. 100) and entered into force on 7 April 1948. The Definition has not been amended since 1948."

16. An excellent analysis of this question can be found in Winston Smith, "Dichotomy or Tricotomy? How the Doctrine of Man Shapes the Treatment of

Depression," *The Journal of Biblical Counseling* 18, no. 3 (Spring 2000): 21–29. Although we differ with Smith's ultimate conclusions as they apply to treating depression because they are inconsistent with his own view that man is inseparably material and immaterial (our view is that man is a biopsychosociospiritual entity), we recommend his exposition of related Scriptures and his analysis of the book *Happiness Is a Choice*.

17. Harold G. Koenig, James Blumenthal, and K. Moore, "New Version of Brief Depression Scale," *Journal of the American Geriatrics Society* 43 (1995): 1447 (reprinted with permission).

Chapter 3. Do Real Christians Get Depressed?

1. J. B. Phillips, *Your God Is Too Small* (New York: Simon and Schuster/Touchstone, 1997), 30.

2. J. B. Phillips, *The Price of Success* (Wheaton, Ill.: Harold Shaw, 1984), 197.

3. Ibid., 200–202.

4. Jan Dravecky, *A Joy I'd Never Known: One Woman's Triumph over Panic Attacks and Depression* (Grand Rapids: Zondervan, 1996), 119–20.

5. Dr. Koenig's story is told most effectively in the first part of his book, *The Healing Connection* (Nashville: Word, 2000).

6. Catherine B. Allen, *The New Lottie Moon Story* (Nashville: Broadman, 1980), 100.

7. Ibid., 160.

8. Abraham Lincoln, in his 23 January 1841 letter to John T. Stuart, Lincoln's first law partner.

9. Milton H. Shutes, *Lincoln and the Doctors: A Medical Narrative of the Life of Abraham Lincoln* (New York: Pioneer Press, 1933) and Michael Burlingame, *The Inner World of Abraham Lincoln* (Chicago: University of Illinois Press, 1994), especially chapter 5, "Lincoln's Depressions: 'Melancholy Dript from Him as He Walked.'"

10. Sheila Walsh, *Honestly* (Grand Rapids: Zondervan, 1996), 99–100.

11. H. G. Koenig, D. G. Blazer, G. S. Alexopoulous, ed., "Epidemiology of Geriatric Affective Disorder," *Clinics in Geriatric Medicine* 8 (1992): 235–52.

12. Boris Birmaher, Neil D. Ryan, Douglas E. Williamson, David A. Brent, "Childhood and Adolescent Depression: A Review of the Past 10 Years, Part 1," *Journal of the American Academy of Child and Adolescent Psychiatry* 35 (1996): 1427–39; Peter M. Lewinsohn, Hyman Hops, Robert E. Roberts, John R. Seeley, "Adolescent Psychopathology: I. Prevalence and Incidence of Depression and Other DSM-III-R Disorders in High School Students," *Journal of Abnormal Psychology* 102 (1993): 133–44; Martin B. Keller, Philip W. Lavori, William R. Beardslee, Joanne Wunder, "Depression in Children and Adolescents: New Data on 'Undertreatment' and a Literature Review on the Efficacy of Available Treatments," *Journal of Affective Disorders* 21 (1991): 163–71; Paul Rohde, Peter M. Lewinsohn, and John R. Seeley, "Comorbidity of Unipolar Depression: II. Comorbidity with Other Mental Disorders in Adolescents and Adults," *Journal of Abnormal Psychology* 100 (1991): 214–22.

13. National Mental Health Association: *http://www.nmha.org*.

14. Adapted from George Nichols and David Biebel, "Do Real Christians Get Depressed?" *Today's Christian Doctor*, HealthWise special edition (Fall 1995): 8–10. Used by permission.

15. Ibid., revised with new life-saving questions © David B. Biebel, 2004.

Chapter 4. Ten Myths and Misconceptions

1. Arnold A. Dallimore, *Spurgeon: A New Biography* (Carlisle, Pa.: Banner of Truth Trust, 1987), 186.

2. The "five essential characteristics" of addiction are described in Gerald G. May, *Addiction and Grace* (New York: Harper and Row, 1988), 26–30. Note that his list is not as long as the list associated with the World Health Organization's description of *dependence* (another word for *addiction*). The WHO's list is, in summary: 1. Strong desire or sense of compulsion; 2. Difficulty in controlling; 3. Withdrawal pain or anxiety; 4. Use of a similar substance to avoid the symptoms of withdrawal; 5. Increased tolerance; 6. Neglect of alternative pleasures or interests.

3. Ibid., 28.

4. From "Meditation XVII," in *Devotions upon Emergent Occasions* (1625).

5. Dwight Carlson, *Why Do Christians Shoot Their Wounded?* (Downers Grove, Ill.: InterVarsity Press, 1994), 9.

6. See chapter 10.

7. C. H. Spurgeon, *Sermons*, vol. 2, 169–70, cited in Skoglund, *Bright Days, Dark Nights*, 84.

8. See our final chapter for more on this theme.

9. John White, *The Masks of Melancholy* (Downers Grove, Ill.: InterVarsity Press, 1982), 202–3.

10. Jack L. Arnold, "Martin Luther: From Birth to Conversion (1463–1516)," *IIIM Magazine Online*, 1, no. 3, (15–21 March 1999), *www.thirdmill.org/files/english/html/ch/CH.Arnold.RMT.3.HTML.*

11. Biographical material based on the book by Norman E. Nygaard, *A Mighty Fortress—the Life of Martin Luther* (Grand Rapids: Zondervan, 1964).

12. See 1 Thessalonians 4:13–18, here summarized according to its meaning in the original Greek.

13. Dravecky, *A Joy I'd Never Known*, 136–37.

14. Phillips, *The Price of Success*, 205.

15. St. John of the Cross, *The Dark Night of the Soul*, 97–98.

Chapter 5. Strategies and Pitfalls for Those Who Wish to Help Themselves

1. This is the primary message of 1 Corinthians 12–14.

2. This is the primary point of Romans 14:1–4, "Accept him whose faith is weak, without passing judgment on disputable matters. . . . Who are you to judge someone else's servant? To his own master he stands or falls. And he will stand, for the Lord is able to make him stand."

3. "Life coaching" is a relatively new movement in which a "coach" helps a "client" identify goals and objectives and stay on track toward achieving these. As such, life coaching is not psychotherapy in a strict sense, though it employs certain psychological principles apparently related to the central tenets of William Glasser's "reality therapy" (1960s), which is based on "choice theory." Information on life coaching and reality therapy/choice therapy can be found online at: *http://www.lifecoaching.com* and *http://www.wglasser.com.*

4. J. H. McHenry, *Prayer Walk: Becoming a Woman of Prayer, Strength, and Discipline* (Colorado Springs: Waterbrook Press, 2001).

5. Richard A. Swenson, *Margin* (Colorado Springs: NavPress, 1992), and Richard A. Swenson, *The Overload Syndrome* (Colorado Springs: NavPress, 1998).

6. Dónal O'Mathúna and Walt Larimore, *Alternative Medicine: The Christian Handbook* (Grand Rapids: Zondervan, 2001).

7. Jonathan R. T. Davidson, et al., "Effect of Hypericum Perforatum (St John's Wort) in Major Depressive Disorder, a Randomized Controlled Trial," *Journal of the American Medical Association* 287, no.14 (2002): 1807–14.

8. *New Man* (Jan./Feb. 1997), 44–48. Used by permission.

9. See the web site: *http://www.stonegateresources.org.* See also Harry Schaumburg, *False Intimacy*, rev. ed. (Colorado Springs: NavPress, 1997).

10. Contact information for Dr. McBurney: Marble Retreat, 139 Bamrockburn, Marble, Colorado, 81623. Telephone (970) 963-2499. *Http://www.marbleretreat.org.*

11. This list is not exhaustive. Psychosomatic symptoms are as varied as the people who have them. Only careful medical evaluation can sort it out.

12. See chapter 8 for an example of this.

Chapter 6. Mental Health Professionals

1. We use the words *licensed* and *certified* interchangeably because they mean essentially the same thing.

2. *http://www.counseling.org/.*

3. Marriage and Family Therapists (MFTs) often employ theory and methods from various schools of psychotherapy as appropriate to the client. Most use a "holistic" approach, considering the person's biological, psychological, sociological, and spiritual needs and issues. For some MFTs, the word *spiritual* is far less defined than it would be when used by a Christian, so believers seeking help from MFTs may wish to clarify in advance a particular therapist's perspective on spirituality. For more information on MFTs, consult the web site *www.aamft.org.*

4. *http://www.aacc.net/index.html?main=aboutaacc.html.*
5. *http://www.aapc.org/.*
6. *http://www.apa.org/.*
7. *http://www.caps.net./*
8. *http://www.psych.org/.*
9. *http://www.actheals.org/.*
10. Various counseling approaches are explained in chapters 7 and 8.
11. Electroconvulsive therapy (ECT) is described more fully in chapter 10.
12. See chapter 10 for more detailed information about bipolar disorder and its treatments.
13. A form to help you prepare for your initial consultation with a mental health professional can be found at the end of this chapter.
14. Adapted from David L. Stevens, "How to Talk to Your Doctor," *Today's Christian Doctor,* HealthWise special edition (Spring/Summer 1996): 26–27. Used by permission.

Chapter 7. Counseling Models and Methods

1. J. B. Persons, M. E. Thase, P. Crits-Christoph, "The Role of Psychotherapy in the Treatment of Depression: Review of Two Practice Guidelines," *Archives of General Psychiatry* 53 (1996): 283–90. M. E. Thase et al., "Treatment of Major Depression with Psychotherapy or Psychotherapy-Pharmacotherapy Combinations," *Archives of General Psychiatry* 54 (1997): 1009–15. Bear in mind that the latter statements apply only to psychotherapies that have been studied in clinical trial (mostly interpersonal psychotherapy and cognitive or behavioral psychotherapy). It is unwise to generalize this finding to all forms of counseling, which do vary in their effectiveness.
2. See the end of the chapter for suggestions about how to choose a therapist.
3. The session dialogues are fictitious. Any similarity to persons living or dead is coincidental.
4. Cecilia Capuzzi Simon, "A Change of Mind: Thanks to Managed Care, Evidence-Based Medical Practice and Changing Ideas about Behavior, Cognitive Therapy Is the Talking Cure of the Moment," *Washington Post,* 3 September 2002, HE01.
5. This theory is theoretically connected with the field of cybernetics (from the Greek: "the science of governance or control"). Family systems theory should not be confused with psycho-cybernetics (a la Maxwell Maltz; i.e., "mind-control"), which implies that by an exercise of your mind you can control what happens (become the master of your own destiny). Within the Christian worldview, God controls what happens, and he is the ultimate master of our destiny. Family systems theory can be helpful when trying to understand and counsel a family in distress, as it tries for an integrative approach that considers various perspectives, including the perspectives of the children.
6. See the dreamweaving checklist at the end of this chapter.
7. Sigmund Freud, "Mourning and Melancholia," in *General Psychological Theory,* vol. 5 of *Sigmund Freud: Collected Papers,* ed. Philip Riett (New York: Collier, 1917), 165.
8. White, *Masks of Melancholy,* 106.

Chapter 8. Models and Methods of Christian Counseling

1. *Nondirective* counseling reflects back to the client what the client has said or felt. For example, had LezLee said she was really angry that the highway's condition had contributed to Nicholle's death, the counselor might respond, "You feel angry because the road condition was so poor."
2. This would be an example of a more directive approach, in which the counselor advises or strongly encourages the client to do or not do something or to view a situation or problem in a particular way.
3. By *general* we mean not associated with or affiliated with any particular school of psychology, theology, or counseling methodology.
4. This is most likely an interactive counselor, who listens well, asks questions to lead to better insights and/or decisions, and gives advice or direction as needed.
5. LezLee is sharing her story nationwide and many people are being blessed. She is pursuing her vision to provide a resting place in the Colorado Rocky Mountains where bereaved parents can come and find support, understanding, love, and ultimately healing. To learn more about Sunshyne Ministries, call (719) 548–8917.

6. W. Backus and M. Chapin, *Telling Yourself the Truth* (Minneapolis: Bethany House, 2000). F. O'Shields, *Slaying the Giant: Practical Help for Understanding, Preventing, and Overcoming Depression* (Surfside Beach, S.C.: Hem of His Garment Publishers, 1995).

7. Gary Collins, *Overcoming Anxiety* (Santa Ana, Calif.: Vision House, 1973), 8.

8. Gary Collins, *Christian Counseling: A Comprehensive Guide* (Nashville: Word, 1988).

9. *http://www.aacc.net/.*

10. *http://www.ncca-usa.com/home.html.*

11. *http://www.aactonline.net/.*

12. *http://www.nanc.org/nancWHATISNOUTHETIC COUSELING.shtml.*

13. Martin Bobgan and Diedre Bobgan, *Prophets of Psychoheresy* (Santa Barbara, Calif.: EastGate Publishers, 1989).

14. See Miles J. Stanford's piece titled "Incompetent to Counsel" at *http://www.rapidnet.com/~jbeard/bdm/exposes/macarthur/counseli.htm.*

15. Jay E. Adams, *Competent to Counsel* (Phillipsburg, N.J.: Presbyterian and Reformed Publishing Company, 1974), 97–99.

16. Ibid., 125–26.

17. The entire section (2 Peter 1:3–11) has great relevance to how a Christian can build a depression-resistant life.

18. *http://www.restcounseling.com/rest.html.*

19. *http://www.theophostic.com/.*

20. Note that the translation of this phrase could just as easily be: "I will be who I will be."

21. See 1 Corinthians 12–14, with all its creative imagery, for Paul's extended discussion of the body and its parts.

22. *http://www.hope-healing.com/.*

Chapter 9. Antidepressant Medications

1. See Debbie Thurman, *From Depression to Wholeness* (Monroe, Va.: Cedar House Publishers, 2000).

2. "Practice Guidelines for the Treatment of Patients with Major Depressive Disorder," revision, *American Journal of Psychiatry* 157, supplement (2000): 1–45.

3. Note to counselors: All counselors (including clergy who do psychotherapy) should encourage their clinically depressed clients to have a thorough medical evaluation not only to obtain pharmacological treatment for the depression but also to rule out other possible causes such as hypothyroidism. Therapists, including clergy, may be at risk for a malpractice suit if one of their depressed counselees, who is not also being treated with antidepressant medication, commits suicide. The family may claim that the therapist should have insisted that the depressed person seek a medical evaluation and treatment since treatment with antidepressants is the standard of treatment for clinical depression. Christian counselors who believe they should discourage depressed patients who are not already on antidepressants from beginning such treatment would be wise to get some good legal advice about how to ensure that the patient and family are fully informed.

4. A. Khan, R. M. Leventhal, S. R. Khan, W. A. Brown, "Severity of Depression and Response to Antidepressants and Placebo: An Analysis of the Food and Drug Administration Database," *Journal of Clinical Psychopharmacology* 22, no. 1 (2000): 40–45.

5. The dosages used here are equivalent.

6. This is not intended as a comprehensive list of side effects but only to describe the kinds of side effects likely to be encountered.

7. The information in this section is based on norms and not intended to replace or challenge your doctor's plan of medication for you, which should be personalized to address your specific needs.

8. Roper Reports, *To Medicate: What People Do for Minor Health Problems* (New York: Roper Organization, October 1986), 86–88.

9. Gary Langer, "Use of Anti-depressants Is a Long-Term Practice" (10 April 2000). Available at: *http://more.abcnews.go.com/onair/dailynews/poll000410.html.*

10. Olfson et al., "National Trends in the Outpatient Treatment of Depression," 203–9.

11. See the section "Straight Talk with Your Doctor" at the end of this chapter.

Chapter 10. Other Treatments for Depression

1. See the end of the chapter for a list of other medications for depression besides antidepressants.

2. © Copyright, Cherish, Inc.

3. In psychiatric terms, *acute hospitalization* is admission to a psychiatric unit in a general hospital. *Chronic hospitalization,* by contrast, means admission to a state hospital, mental institution, nursing home, or other long-term care facility.

4. R. M. Glass, "Electroconvulsive Therapy: Time to Bring It out of the Shadow," *Journal of the American Medical Association* 285, no. 10 (2001): 1346–48.

5. A. McDonald, G. Walter, "The Portrayal of ECT in American Movies," *Journal of ECT* 17, no. 4 (2001): 264–74.

6. A. B. Donahue, "Electroconvulsive Therapy and Memory Loss: A Personal Journey," *Journal of ECT* 16, no. 2 (2000): 133–43.

7. D. P. Devanand et al., "Does ECT Alter Brain Structure?" *American Journal of Psychiatry* 151, no. 7 (1994): 957–70.

8. Glass, "Electroconvulsive Therapy," 1346–48.

9. B. J. Saddock, V. A. Saddock, *Comprehensive Textbook of Psychiatry*, 7th ed. (New York: Lippincott Williams and Wilkins, 2000), 3109.

10. A. J. P. Gregoire et al., "Transdermal Estrogen for Treatment of Severe Postnatal Depression," *Lancet* 347 (1996): 930–33.

11. A. Ahokas et al., "Estrogen Deficiency in Severe Postpartum Depression," *Journal of Clinical Psychiatry* 62 (2001): 332–36.

12. L. J. Miller, "Postpartum Depression," *Journal of the American Medical Association* 287, no. 6 (2002): 762–65.

13. U. Halbreich, "Role of Estrogen in Postmenopausal Depression," *Neurology* 48, no. 5, Supplement 7 (1997): 16S–20S.

14. Claudio de Novaes Soares et al., "Efficacy of Estradiol for the Treatment of Depressive Disorders in Perimenopausal Women: A Double-Blind, Randomized, Placebo-Controlled Trial," *Archives of General Psychiatry* 58, no. 6 (2001): 529–34.

15. M. S. George et al., "Mood Improvement Following Daily Left Prefrontal Repetitive Magnetic Stimulation in Patients with Depression: A Placebo-Controlled Crossover Trial," *American Journal of Psychiatry* 154 (1997): 1752–56.

16. For a report on this clinical trial, see the web site: *http://www.pslgroup.com/dg/15131a.htm.*

17. Even secular authors use such terminology to describe depression, as in Solomon, *Noonday Demon.*

18. John Warwick Montgomery, ed., *Demon Possession* (Minneapolis: Bethany Fellowship, 1976).

19. White, *Masks of Melancholy*, 30–31.

20. Methods similar to these were described in David Seamands, *Healing for Damaged Emotions* (Wheaton, Ill.: Victor, 1981), and David Seamands, *Healing of Memories* (Wheaton, Ill.: Victor, 1985).

Chapter 11. Love

1. Solomon, *Noonday Demon*, 15.

2. Laura Epstein Rosen and Xavier Francisco Amador, *When Someone You Love Is Depressed: How to Help Your Loved One without Losing Yourself* (New York: Simon and Schuster, 1997), 146.

3. This phrase is used repeatedly by Rosen and Amador, *When Someone You Love Is Depressed.*

4. For an extended discussion of these dynamics and how to constructively overcome them, see Rosen and Amador, *When Someone You Love Is Depressed,* 147–62.

5. I (DB) take this to be the meaning of Ephesians 4:8–9, specifically that through his life, death, resurrection, and ascension, Jesus defeated Satan and conquered death by taking the curse of sin (and all things related to it) upon himself. As a result, God grants everlasting life to all who believe in Jesus (John 3:16).

6. Mitch Golant and Susan K. Golant, *What to Do When Someone You Love Is Depressed* (New York: Henry Holt and Company, 1996), 3–4.

7. From Merriam-Webster On-Line: *http://www.webster.com/.*

8. White, *Masks of Melancholy*, 141.

9. Don Baker and Emery Nester, *Depression: Finding Hope and Meaning in Life's Darkest Shadow* (Portland, Ore.: Multnomah Press, 1983).

10. Timothy J. Demy and Gary P. Stewart, eds., *Suicide: A Christian Response* (Grand Rapids: Kregel Publications, 1998).

11. It is hard to define the term *mentally ill.* In this case, the author of the original list seems to be limiting its meaning to "psychotic," since depression is thought by most secular writers to be an illness of the mind (thus "mental illness"). However, in this

book we have used a much broader definition of depression; specifically, that it is a state of existence marked by a sense of being pressed down, weighed down, or burdened, which affects a person physically, mentally, spiritually, and relationally. Therefore, it is not a state of mind (i.e., not an illness of the mind, per se), but a state of *being*.

12. In *Masks of Melancholy*, 164–68, Dr. White lists eight fables and facts about suicide and then adds one of his own. The first eight are based on E. S. Schneidman, "Suicide," *Comprehensive Textbook of Psychiatry*, A. M. Freedman, H. I. Kaplan, and B. J. Sadock, eds. (Baltimore: Williams and Wilkins Co., 1975), 174–85. This list is adapted from the above; the tenth fable and fact is ours.

13. Albert Camus, *The Myth of Sisyphus and Other Essays*, as quoted in William Styron, *Darkness Visible: A Memoir of Madness* (New York: Random House, 1990), 23.

14. Rosen and Amador, *When Someone You Love Is Depressed*, 177–99.

15. David A. Brent and Boris Birmaher, "Adolescent Depression," *New England Journal of Medicine* 347, no. 9 (29 August 2002): 667–71.

16. Ibid.

17. Styron, *Darkness Visible*, 52–53.

Chapter 12. Faith

1. Peter Kreeft, *Making Sense out of Suffering* (Ann Arbor, Mich.: Servant Books, 1986), 169–70.

2. The impact of attachments on one's mental health is a key concept in *object-relations theory*. In this view, the source of many adult psychological problems is childhood loss. This may relate to what we've called *developmental depression*. Yet a sense of loss as a result of detachments in adulthood can also contribute significantly to depression, whether situational or spiritual, any of which will result in depletion of neurotransmitters over time.

3. Styron, *Darkness Visible*, 57.

4. Jeffery Smith, *Where the Roots Reach for Water* (New York: North Point Press, 1999), 272–74.

5. Frederich Flach, *The Secret Strength of Depression* (New York: Hatherleigh Press, 1995), 17–18.

6. Søren Kierkegaard, quoted by Kreeft, *Making Sense out of Suffering*, 75.

7. Walsh, *Honestly*, 185–87.

8. Debbie Thurman, personal correspondence with David Biebel (21 August 2002).

9. Peter Kreeft, personal correspondence with David Biebel (1987).

10. We'll have more to say about hope in the final chapter.

Chapter 13. Hope

1. C. H. Spurgeon, *Sermons*, vol. 18 (New York: Funk and Wagnalls, n.d.), 351–52.

2. Biebel, *If God Is So Good*, 146.

3. Styron, *Darkness Visible*, 84.

4. Viktor Frankl, *Man's Search for Meaning* (New York: Washington Square Press, 1959), 60.

5. Ibid., 98.

6. Dante Alighieri, *The Divine Comedy: Inferno [Hell]* Canto 34.

7. Harold G. Koenig, James Blumenthal, and K. Moore, "New Version of Brief Depression Scale." *Journal of the American Geriatrics Society* 43 (1995): 1447 (reprinted with permission).

Bibliography

Articles/Periodicals

Ahokas, Antti, Jutta Kaukoranta, Kristian Wahlbeck, and Marjatta Aito. "Estrogen Deficiency in Severe Postpartum Depression." *Journal of Clinical Psychiatry* 62 (2001): 332–36.

Birmaher, Boris, Neal D. Ryan, Douglas E. Williamson, and David A. Brent. "Childhood and Adolescent Depression: A Review of the Past 10 Years, Part I." *Journal of the American Academy of Child and Adolescent Psychiatry* 35 (1996): 1427–39.

Brent, David A., and Boris Birmaher. "Adolescent Depression." *New England Journal of Medicine* 347, no. 9 (29 August 2002): 667–71.

Browder, E. J. "Techniques of Psychosurgery: Report of the Committee on Surgery." *Proceedings of the Third Research Conference on Psychosurgery,* edited by F. A. Mettler, W. Overholser. Public Health Service Publication 221 (Washington, D.C.: U.S. Government Printing Office, 1954).

Devanand, Devangere P., Andrew J. Dwork, Edward R. Hutchinson, Tom G. Bolwig, and Harold A. Sackeim. "Does ECT Alter Brain Structure?" *American Journal of Psychiatry* 151, no. 7 (1994): 957–70.

Donahue, Anne B. "Electroconvulsive Therapy and Memory Loss: A Personal Journey." *Journal of ECT* 16, no. 2 (2000): 133–43.

Feldman, Robert P., and James T. Goodrich. "Psychosurgery: A Historical Overview." *Neurosurgery* 48, no. 3 (2001): 647–59.

George, Mark S., Eric M. Wasserman, Timothy A. Kimbrell, John T. Little, Wendol E. Williams, Aimee L. Danielson, Benjamin D. Greenberg, Mark Hallett, and Robert M. Post. "Mood Improvement Following Daily Left Prefrontal Repetitive Magnetic Stimulation in Patients with Depression: A Placebo-Controlled Crossover Trial." *American Journal of Psychiatry* 154 (1997): 1752–56.

Glass, Richard M. "Electroconvulsive Therapy: Time to Bring It out of the Shadow." *Journal of the American Medical Association* 285, no. 10 (2001): 1346–48.

Gregoire, A. J. P., R. Kumar, B. Everitt, and J. W. Studd. "Transdermal Estrogen for Treatment of Severe Postnatal Depression." *Lancet* 347 (1996): 930–33.

Halbreich, Uriel. "Role of Estrogen in Postmenopausal Depression." *Neurology* 48, no. 5, Supplement 7 (1997): 16S–20S.

Kaelber, Charles T. "Depression and Spirituality." *Health and Spirituality Connection* 5, no. 4 (Winter 2002): 1, 6, 7.

Keller, Martin B., Philip W. Lavori, William R. Beardslee, and Joanne Wunder. "Depression in Children and Adolescents: New Data on 'Undertreatment' and a Literature Review on the Efficacy of Available Treatments." *Journal of Affective Disorders* 21 (1991): 163–71.

Keller, Martin B., James P. McCullough, Daniel N. Klein, Bruce Arnow, David L. Dunner, Alan J. Gelenberg, John C. Markowitz, Charles B. Nemeroff, James M. Russell, Michael E. Thase, Madhukar H. Trivedi, and John Zajecka. "A Comparison of Nefazadone, the Cognitive-Behavioral Analysis System of Psychotherapy, and their Combination for the Treatment of Chronic Depression." *New England Journal of Medicine* 342 (2000): 1462–70.

Kessler, Ronald C., Katharine A. McGonagle, Shanyang Zhao, and Christopher B. Nelson. "Lifetime and 12-Month Prevalence of DSM-III-R Psychiatric Disorders in the United States: Results from the National Comorbidity Survey." *Archives of General Psychiatry* 51 (1994): 8–19.

Khan, Arif, Robyn M. Leventhal, Shirin R. Khan, and Walter A. Brown. "Severity of Depression and Response to Antidepressants and Placebo: An Analysis of the Food and Drug Administration Database." *Journal of Clinical Psychopharmacology* 22, no. 1 (2000): 40–45.

Koenig, Harold G., and Dan G. Blazer. "Epidemiology of Geriatric Affective Disorder." *Clinics in Geriatric Medicine* 8 (1992): 235–52.

Langer, Gary. "Use of Antidepressants Is a Long-Term Practice" (10 April 2000). Available at: *http://more.abcnews.go.com/onair/dailynews/poll0004 10.html.*

Lewinsohn, Peter M., Hyman Hops, Robert E. Roberts, and John R. Seeley. "Adolescent Psychopathology: I. Prevalence and Incidence of Depression and Other DSM-III-R Disorders in High School Students." *Journal of Abnormal Psychology* 102 (1993): 133–44.

McDonald, A., and G. Walter. "The Portrayal of ECT in American Movies." *Journal of ECT* 17, no. 4 (2001): 264–74.

Miller, Laura J. "Postpartum Depression." *Journal of the American Medical Association* 287, no. 6 (2002): 762–65.

Morrow, D. J. "Lusting after Prozac." *New York Times* (11 October 1998), section 3, 1, 8.

Nichols, George, and David Biebel. "Do Real Christians Get Depressed?" *Today's Christian Doctor,* HealthWise special edition (Fall 1995).

Olfson, Mark, Steven C. Marcus, Benjamin Druss, Lynn Elinson, Terri Tanielian, and Harold Alan Pincus. "National Trends in the Outpatient Treatment of Depression." *Journal of the American Medical Association* 287 (2002): 203–9.

Persons, Jacqueline B., Michael E. Thase, and Paul Crits-Christoph. "The Role of Psychotherapy in the Treatment of Depression: Review of Two Practice Guidelines." *Archives of General Psychiatry* 53 (1996): 283–90.

"Practice Guidelines for the Treatment of Patients with Major Depressive Disorder," revision. *American Journal of Psychiatry* 157, supplement (2000): 1–45.

Regier, Darrel A., William E. Narrow, Donald S. Rae, Ronald W. Manderscheid, Ben Z. Locke, and Fred K. Goodwin. "The De Facto US Mental and Addictive Disorders Service System: Epidemiologic Catchment Area Prospective 1-Year Prevalence Rates of Disorders and Services." *Archives of General Psychiatry* 50 (1993): 85–94.

Rohde, Paul, Peter M. Lewinsohn, and John R. Seeley. "Comorbidity of Unipolar Depression: II. Comorbidity with Other Mental Disorders in Adolescents and Adults." *Journal of Abnormal Psychology* 100 (1991): 214–22.

Smith, Winston. "Dichotomy or Tricotomy? How the Doctrine of Man Shapes the Treatment of Depression." *The Journal of Biblical Counseling* 18, no. 3 (Spring 2000): 21–29.

Soares, Claudio de Novaes, Osvaldo P. Almeida, Hadine Joffe, and Lee S. Cohen. "Efficacy of Estradiol for the Treatment of Depressive Disorders in Perimenopausal Women: A Double-Blind, Randomized, Placebo-Controlled Trial." *Archives of General Psychiatry* 58, no. 6 (2001): 529–34.

"Spirit of the Age: Malignant Sadness Is the World's Great Hidden Burden." *The Economist*, editorial (19 December 1998): 113–17.

Steffens, David C., Ingrid Svenson, Douglas A. Marchuk, Robert M. Levy, Judith C. Hays, Elizabeth P. Flint, K. Ranga Rama Krishnan, and Ilene C. Siegler. "Allelic Differences in the Serotonin Transport-Linked Polymorphic Region in Geriatric Depression." *American Journal of Geriatric Psychiatry* 10, no. 2 (2002): 185–91.

Stevens, David L. "How to Talk to Your Doctor." *Today's Christian Doctor* (Spring/Summer 1996, HealthWise special edition): 26–27.

Thase, Michael E., Joel B. Greenhouse, Ellen Frank, Charles F. Reynolds III, Paul A. Pilkonis, Katharine Hurley, Victoria Grochocinski, and David J. Kupfer. "Treatment of Major Depression with Psychotherapy or Psychotherapy-Pharmacotherapy Combinations." *Archives of General Psychiatry* 54 (1997): 1009–15.

Books

Adams, Jay E. *Competent to Counsel*. Phillipsburg, N.J.: Presbyterian and Reformed Publishing Co., 1970.

Allen, Catherine B. *The New Lottie Moon Story*. Nashville: Broadman Press, 1980.

American Psychiatric Association. *Diagnostic and Manual of Mental Disorders,* 4th ed. Washington, D.C.: APA Press, 1994.

Backus, W., and M. Chapin. *Telling Yourself the Truth*. Minneapolis: Bethany House, 2000.

Baker, Don, and Emery Nester. *Depression: Finding Hope and Meaning in Life's Darkest Shadow*. Portland, Ore.: Multnomah Press, 1983.

Bernall, Misty. *She Said Yes—The Unlikely Martyrdom of Cassie Bernall*. New York: Simon and Schuster, 1999.

Biebel, David B. *How to Help a Heartbroken Friend*. Grand Rapids: Revell, 1993.

———. *If God Is So Good, Why Do I Hurt So Bad?* Grand Rapids: Baker, 1995.

———. *Jonathan, You Left Too Soon*. Old Tappan, N.J.: Revell, 1997.

Bobgan, Martin M., and Diedre Bobgan. *Prophets of Psychoheresy I*. Santa Barbara, Calif.: EastGate Publishers, 1989.

Brand, Paul, and Philip Yancey. *Pain: The Gift Nobody Wants*. New York: HarperCollins, 1993.

Bunyan, John. *The Pilgrim's Progress*. Nashville: Thomas Nelson, 1999 edition.

Burlingame, Michael. *The Inner World of Abraham Lincoln*. Chicago: University of Illinois Press, 1994.

Burton, Robert. *The Anatomy of Melancholy*. New York: New York Review of Books, 2001.

Camus, Albert. *The Myth of Sisyphus and Other Essays*. New York: Knopf, 1955.

Carlson, Dwight. *Why Do Christians Shoot Their Wounded?* Downers Grove, Ill.: InterVarsity Press, 1994.

Chave-Jones, Myra. *Coping with Depression*. Bellevelle, Mich.: Lion Publishing Corp., 1981.

Christenson, Evelyn. *Gaining through Losing*. Wheaton, Ill.: Victor, 1980.

Collins, Gary. *Overcoming Anxiety*. Santa Ana, Calif.: Vision House, 1973.

Csikszentmihalyi, Mihaly. *Creativity*. New York: HarperCollins, 1996.

Dallimore, Arnold. *Spurgeon: A New Biography*. Carlisle, Pa.: Banner of Truth Trust, 1985.

Demy, Timothy J., and Gary P. Stewart, eds. *Suicide: A Christian Response*. Grand Rapids: Kregel Publications, 1998.

Dravecky, Jan. *A Joy I'd Never Known: One Woman's Triumph over Panic Attacks and Depression*. Grand Rapids: Zondervan, 1996.

Fenelon. *Let Go*. Springdale, Pa.: Whitaker House, 1973.

Flach, Frederich. *The Secret Strength of Depression*. New York: Hatherleigh Press, 1995.

Frankl, Viktor E. *Man's Search for Meaning*. New York: Washington Square Press, 1959.

Frey, William C. *The Dance of Hope*. Colorado Springs: Waterbrook Press, 2003.

Golant, Mitch, and Susan K. Golant. *What to Do When Someone You Love Is Depressed*. New York: Henry Holt and Company, 1996.

Graham, Billy. *Unto the Hills: A Daily Devotional*. Dallas: Word, 1996.

Graham, Ruth Bell. *Prodigals and Those Who Love Them*. Grand Rapids: Baker, 1999.

Jamison, Kay Redfield. *Touched with Fire*. New York: Simon and Schuster, 1993.

———. *An Unquiet Mind*. New York: Alfred A. Knopf, 1995.

John of the Cross. *The Dark Night of the Soul*. New York: Doubleday, 1990.

Kierkegaard, Søren. *Fear and Trembling* and *The Sickness unto Death,* trans. Walter Lowrie. Princeton, N.J.: Princeton University Press, 1941.

Koenig, Harold G. *The Healing Connection.* Nashville: Word, 2000.

———. *Purpose and Power in Retirement: New Opportunities for Meaning and Significance.* Philadelphia: Templeton Foundation Press, 2002.

Kreeft, Peter. *Making Sense out of Suffering.* Ann Arbor, Mich.: Servant Books, 1986.

Lewis, C. S. *The Four Loves.* London and Glasgow: Collins Fontana Books, 1970.

———. *A Grief Observed.* New York: The Seabury Press, 1961.

———. *Mere Christianity.* New York: Macmillan, 1943.

———. *The Problem of Pain.* London and Glasgow: Fontana, 1940.

Luciani, Joseph J. *Self-Coaching—How to Heal Anxiety and Depression.* New York: Jon Wiley and Sons, 2001.

May, Gerald G. *Addiction and Grace.* New York: Harper and Row, 1988.

McHenry, Janet Holm. *Prayer Walk: Becoming a Woman of Prayer, Strength, and Discipline.* Colorado Springs: Waterbrook Press, 2001.

Meier, Paul, and Frank Minirth. *Happiness Is a Choice.* Grand Rapids: Baker, 1994.

Mettler, F. A., and W. Overholser, eds. *Proceedings of the Third Research Conference on Psychosurgery.* Washington, D.C.: U.S. Government Printing Office, 1954.

Miles, Donald G. *Understanding Depression.* Chattanooga, Tenn.: Turning Point Ministries.

Montgomery, John Warwick, ed. *Demon Possession.* Minneapolis: Bethany Fellowship, 1976.

Murray, C., and A. Lopez, *The Global Burden of Disease: A Comprehensive Assessment of Mortality and Disability from Diseases, Injuries, and Risk Factors in 1990 and Projected to 2020.* Vol. 1. Geneva: World Heath Organization.

Nouwen, Henri J. M. *The Inner Voice of Love: A Journey through Anguish to Freedom.* New York: Doubleday/Random House, 1996.

———. *The Return of the Prodigal Son.* New York: Doubleday, 1994.

———. *The Way of the Heart.* San Francisco: Harper and Row, 1981.

———. *The Wounded Healer.* New York: Doubleday, 1979.

Nygaard, Norman E. *A Mighty Fortress: The Life of Martin Luther.* Grand Rapids: Zondervan, 1964.

O'Connor, Richard. *Undoing Depression: What Therapy Doesn't Teach You and Medication Can't Give You.* Rev. ed. New York: Berkley Books, 1999.

O'Mathúna, Dónal, and Walt Larimore. *Alternative Medicine: The Christian Handbook.* Grand Rapids: Zondervan, 2001.

O'Shields, French. *Slaying the Giant: Practical Help for Understanding, Preventing, and Overcoming Depression.* Surfside Beach, S.C.: Hem of His Garment Publishers, 1994.

Pearce, Gillian. *7 Steps to a Depression Free Life: A Self Help Guide.* http://www.depression-recovery-life.com/ebook.html.

Phillips, J. B. *The Price of Success.* Wheaton, Ill.: Harold Shaw, 1984.

———. *Your God Is Too Small.* New York: Simon and Shuster, Inc., 1997.

Piper, John. *The Hidden Smile of God: The Fruit of Affliction in the Lives of John Bunyan, William Cowper, and David Brainerd.* Wheaton, Ill.: Crossway Books, 2001.

Real, Terrence. *I Don't Want to Talk about It.* New York: Simon and Schuster/Fireside, 1998.

Roper Reports. *To Medicate: What People Do for Minor Health Problems.* New York: Roper Organization, 1986.

Rosen, Laura Epstein, and Xavier Francisco Amador. *When Someone You Love Is Depressed: How to Help Your Loved One without Losing Yourself.* New York: Simon and Schuster, 1997.

Saddock, B. J., and V. A. Saddock, *Comprehensive Textbook of Psychiatry,* 7th ed. New York: Lippincott Williams and Wilkins, 2000.

Schaefer, Edith. *Affliction: A Compassionate Look at the Reality of Pain and Suffering.* Old Tappan, N.J.: Revell, 1978.

Seamands, David. *Healing for Damaged Emotions.* Wheaton, Ill.: Victor, 1981.

———. *Healing of Memories.* Wheaton, Ill.: Victor, 1985.

Shields, C., and C. Ferrell. *Spiritual Survival Guide: How to Find God When You're Sick.* New York: Doubleday, 2001.

Skoglund, Elizabeth Ruth. *Bright Days, Dark Nights: With Charles Spurgeon in Triumph over Emotional Pain*. Grand Rapids: Baker, 2000.

Smedes, Lewis B. *Shame and Grace*. San Francisco: Harper/Zondervan, 1993.

Smith, Jeffery. *Where the Roots Reach for Water*. New York: North Point Press, 1999.

Solomon, Andrew. *The Noonday Demon: An Atlas of Depression*. New York: Scribner, 2001.

Spurgeon, C. H. *Sermons*. New York: Funk and Wagnalls, n.d. (cited in Skoglund, *Bright Days, Dark Nights*).

Storr, Anthony. *Churchill's Black Dog, Kafka's Mice*. New York: Ballentine Books, 1965.

Styron, William. *Darkness Visible: A Memoir of Madness*. New York: Random House, 1990.

Swenson, Richard A. *Margin*. Colorado Springs: NavPress, 1992.

———. *The Overload Syndrome*. Colorado Springs: NavPress, 1998.

Tada, Joni Eareckson, and S. Estes. *When God Weeps: Why Our Sufferings Matter to the Almighty*. Grand Rapids: Zondervan, 1996.

Thorne, Julia, with Larry Rothstein. *You Are Not Alone: Words of Experience and Hope for the Journey through Depression*. New York: HarperCollins Publishers, 1993.

Thurman, Debbie. *From Depression to Wholeness*. Monroe, Va.: Cedar House Publishers, 2000.

Tournier, Paul. *Creative Suffering*. San Francisco: Harper and Row, 1983.

———. *The Healing of Persons*. San Francisco: Harper and Row, 1983.

———. *Fatigue in Modern Society*. Atlanta: John Knox Press, 1971.

———. *Guilt and Grace*. San Francisco: Harper and Row, 1983.

———. *The Meaning of Persons*. San Francisco: Harper and Row/Perennial Library, 1973.

———. *The Whole Person in a Broken World*. San Francisco: Harper and Row, 1964.

Walsh, Sheila. *Honestly*. Grand Rapids: Zondervan, 1996.

White, John. *The Masks of Melancholy*. Downers Grove, Ill.: InterVarsity Press, 1982.

Williams, Margery. *The Velveteen Rabbit*. New York: Doubleday/Bantam-Avon Books, 1975.

Winter, D. B. *Closer Than a Brother: Practicing the Presence of God*. Wheaton, Ill.: Harold Shaw, 1971.

Yancey, Philip. *Disappointment with God: Three Questions No One Asks Aloud*. Grand Rapids: Zondervan, 1988.

———. *What's So Amazing about Grace?* Grand Rapids: Zondervan, 1997.

Web Sites and Other Resources

American Association of Christian Counselors: *www.aacc.net*

American Association of Pastoral Counselors: *www.aapc.org*

American Counseling Association: *www.counseling.org*

American Psychiatric Association: *www.psych.org*

America Psychological Association: *www.apa.org*

Association of Christian Therapists: *www.actheals.org*

California State University, "Antidepressants," with diagrams by Keith A. Trujillo, Ph.D.: *www.csusm.edu/psychology/DandB/AD.html*

Center for the Study of Religion/Spirituality and Health, Duke University Medical Center: *www.dukespiritualityandhealth.org*

Christian Association for Psychological Studies: *www.caps.net*

Christian Medical & Dental Associations: *www.cmdahome.org*

Hope Central Ministries: *www.hopecentral.us*

National Institute for Mental Health: *www.nimh.nih.gov*

National Mental Health Association: *www.nmha.org*

Sheila Walsh: *www.sheilawalsh.com*

Index

About the Authors

Dr. Biebel holds the Doctor of Ministry (in Personal Wholeness) from Gordon-Conwell Theological Seminary in South Hamilton, Massachusetts. He has edited the Christian Medical and Dental Associations' flagship journal, *Today's Christian Doctor,* since 1992. Prior to that he edited the *Focus on the Family Physician*. He is an expert on recovery from losses, a speaker at workshops, seminars, and retreats, a frequent radio and television guest, author of many magazine articles, and contributor of several book chapters. He has ghost-authored, coauthored, or otherwise collaborated on seven books, including *Romancing Your Child's Heart* and its manual. He has authored five other books including *Jonathan, You Left Too Soon, How to Help a Heartbroken Friend,* two novels, and the best-seller *If God Is So Good, Why Do I Hurt So Bad?*

Dr. Biebel was raised in New England, where his father was a Baptist minister. The author and his family now live in Colorado, where he enjoys bow hunting, mushrooming, fishing, camping, and otherwise roaming the beautiful Rockies with his wife, Ilona. Dr. Biebel fancies himself a gourmet cook and sometimes refers to himself in the third person, especially when his burnt offerings are suitable only for their English springer spaniel, Brownie.

Dr. Koenig earned his M.D. at the University of California (San Francisco), completing his geriatric medicine, psychiatry, and biostatistics training at Duke University Medical Center. He is board certified in geriatric psychiatry and geriatric medicine and is now on the faculty at Duke as an Associate Professor of Psychiatry and a tenured Associate Professor of Medicine. Dr. Koenig is director and founder of the Center for the

Study of Religion/Spirituality and Health at that institution and has published extensively in the fields of mental health, geriatrics, and religion, with over 180 scientific peer-reviewed articles, 45 book chapters, and 24 books to his credit.

Dr. Koenig is the editor-in-chief of both the *International Journal of Psychiatry in Medicine* and *Research News in Science and Theology*. His research on religion, health, and ethical issues in medicine has been featured on many national and international radio and television news programs and has been highlighted in *Reader's Digest, Prevention Magazine, McCall's, Time Magazine, New York Times, USA Today, Parade, Newsweek*, and many other popular national periodicals. His latest books include *The Healing Power of Faith: Science Explores Medicine's Last Great Frontier* (Simon and Schuster, 1999), *The Healing Connection* (Word Publishers, 2000), and *The Handbook of Religion and Health: A Century of Research Reviewed* (Oxford University Press, 2001). Dr. Koenig has been a guest on *The 700 Club* and on several PAX TV specials. He appeared on James Dobson's radio show (April 17 and 18, 2000) and frequently gives talks to Christian audiences.

Dr. Koenig was raised in Lodi, California, where his father was a vineyardist. Dr. Koenig now lives in Durham, North Carolina, with his wife and children. They attend regularly and are committed to a nondenominational Christian church in Durham.

To contact the authors:

Dr. Biebel: *www.hopecentral.us; dbbv1@aol.com*
Dr. Koenig: *koenig@geri.duke.edu*

Christian
Medical
Association

Resources

Medically reliable . . . biblically sound. That's the rock-solid promise of this series offered by Zondervan in partnership with the Christian Medical Association. Each book in this series is not only written by fully credentialed, experienced doctors but is also fully reviewed by an objective board of qualified doctors to ensure its reliability. Because when your health is at stake, you can't settle for anything less than the whole and accurate truth.

Integrating your faith and health can improve your physical well-being and even extend your life, as you gain insights into the interconnection of health and faith-a relationship largely overlooked by secular science. Benefit from the cutting-edge knowledge of respected medical experts as they help you make health care decisions consistent with your beliefs. Their sound biblical analysis of emerging treatments and technologies equips you to protect yourself from seemingly harmless-yet spiritually, ethically, or medically unsound-options and then to make the healthiest choices possible.

Through this series, you can draw from both the knowledge of science and the wisdom of God's Word in addressing your medical ethics decisions and in meeting your health care needs.

Founded in 1931, the Christian Medical Association helps thousands of doctors minister to their patients by imitating the Great Physician, Jesus Christ. Christian Medical Association members provide a Christian voice on medical ethics to policy makers and the media, minister to needy patients on medical missions around the world, evangelize and disciple students on more than 90 percent of the nation's medical school campuses, and provide educational and inspirational resources to the church.

To learn more about Christian Medical Association ministries and resources on health care and ethical issues, browse the website (www.christianmedicalassociation.org) or call toll-free at 888-231-2637.

"Dear friend, I pray that you may enjoy good health and that all may go well with you, even as your soul is getting along well"(3 John 2 NIV).

We want to hear from you. Please send your comments about this
book to us in care of zreview@zondervan.com. Thank you.

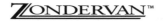

ZONDERVAN™

GRAND RAPIDS, MICHIGAN 49530 USA

WWW.ZONDERVAN.COM